SpringerBriefs in Public Health

SpringerBriefs in Public Health present concise summaries of cutting-edge research and practical applications from across the entire field of public health, with contributions from medicine, bioethics, health economics, public policy, biostatistics, and sociology.

The focus of the series is to highlight current topics in public health of interest to a global audience, including health care policy; social determinants of health; health issues in developing countries; new research methods; chronic and infectious disease epidemics; and innovative health interventions.

Featuring compact volumes of 50 to 125 pages, the series covers a range of content from professional to academic. Possible volumes in the series may consist of timely reports of state-of-the art analytical techniques, reports from the field, snapshots of hot and/or emerging topics, elaborated theses, literature reviews, and in-depth case studies. Both solicited and unsolicited manuscripts are considered for publication in this series.

Briefs are published as part of Springer's eBook collection, with millions of users worldwide. In addition, Briefs are available for individual print and electronic purchase.

Briefs are characterized by fast, global electronic dissemination, standard publishing contracts, easy-to-use manuscript preparation and formatting guidelines, and expedited production schedules. We aim for publication 8-12 weeks after acceptance.

More information about this series at http://www.springer.com/series/10138

Aldo Rosano
Editor

Access to Primary Care and Preventative Health Services of Migrants

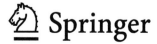 Springer

Editor
Aldo Rosano
National Institute of Health
Rome, Italy

ISSN 2192-3698   ISSN 2192-3701   (electronic)
SpringerBriefs in Public Health
ISBN 978-3-319-73629-7   ISBN 978-3-319-73630-3   (eBook)
https://doi.org/10.1007/978-3-319-73630-3

Library of Congress Control Number: 2018939165

Printed on acid-free paper

This Springer imprint is published by the registered company Springer International Publishing AG part of Springer Nature.
The registered company address is: Gewerbestrasse 11, 6330 Cham, Switzerland

Introduction

Preventive health services (PHS) form part of primary healthcare with the aim of screening for and preventing disease. PHS have a key role in preventing chronic disease, reducing related morbidity and mortality. Preventive healthcare interventions act at different stages of life and may intervene before the occurrence of any disease (primary prevention), or at an early stage of the disease (secondary prevention). Primary prevention includes interventions that aim at preventing the appearance of a disease and include strategies to quit tobacco use, vaccinations/immunization against infectious diseases and health promotion towards healthy lifestyles, including diet and physical activity. Secondary prevention includes activities such as population-based screening programmes for early detection of diseases or provision of chemo-prophylactic agents to control risk factors.

One important piece of preventive strategies relies on health promotion. Health promotion is the process of enabling people to increase control over, and to improve, their health. Health promotion concerns in general diet, physical activity, sexual and reproductive health and healthy lifestyles (WHO 1986).

Migrants show significant differences in lifestyle, health beliefs and risk factors as compared to the native population (Loue and Sajatovic 2012). This could have a significant impact on migrants' access to health systems and participation in prevention programs. On the other hand, barriers to access to preventive health services can be higher than to other health services. Even in countries with widely accessible healthcare systems, migrants' access to preventive health services may be difficult (Mladovsky 2007). Moreover, health promotion programs should be culturally sensitive and adequately targeted in order to reach migrant population and ethnic minorities (Liu 2012).

Nowadays health inequalities are undoubtedly a public health and policy concern. Health care systems are also measured taking into account how equitable they are. The fight against social exclusion could be, in this perspective, a mean of achieving better health care systems. Nevertheless, access to preventive health services is inequitable. "Equity refers to the extent to which access is determined by 'medical need' as proxied by health status as opposed to socio-economic factors such ethnicity, income and insurance status" (Uiters 2009). Gender, socio-economic position and immigrant status have always been the factors analysed to monitor a possible variation in health care access/utilization. There is evidence, although not always coherent, that access to health care services and preventive health services varies between immigrant and native population.

International conventions, such as the International Convenant on Economic, Social and Cultural Rights or the International Convention on the Elimination of All Forms of Racial Discrimination or the Council of Europe Convention on Human Rights and Biomedicine, should ensure equitable access to health care of appropriate quality without any discrimination based on nationality or legal status. Among European countries full access to health care is guaranteed only for migrants in a legal status, with some discrepancies. For undocumented migrants and asylum seekers the situation may vary considerably according to national legislation, as the competence to act in the field of public health is still primarily a national matter (Pace 2011; MIPEX 2017). Major access barriers reported in the literature are lack of awareness of legal entitlements, fear of being reported to authorities, financial obstacles, cultural and language barriers, complexity of actual needs and health problems of the migrant population.

Social determinants may increase the risk of poor health status or poor access to health care services of migrants as the results of a combination of poor social policies and ethnic discrimination.

Access to screening, immunization and treatment is relatively low among undocumented migrants (Chauvin et al. 2009) while one of the main concerns of the receiving countries are infectious diseases surveillance and control such as for HIV, TB and Hepatitis B. Delayed healthcare seeking including the issue of not seeking care at all, cause a deterioration in the health advantage of newly arrived migrants, a possibly more advanced disease at the time of diagnosis and contribute to the invisibility of this population both for registering data and for health services planning. This may induce a bias in the estimation to what extent the access to health services is reduced among migrants.

Data sources of the studies included in the book are mainly health care utilization data, registers and health surveys. Data comparability may be hampered by the heterogeneity in the identification of migrants, the diversity of migrant and ethnic minority groups and the different methods and time of data collection. Nevertheless, it seems possible to carry out cross-country comparisons of health indicators and epidemiologic measures on migrants by using citizenship and/or country of birth, which are available in the majority of health data sources in the European countries (EC 2008).

The book aims at analysing the access to cancer screening programs and vaccination among migrants as well as the access to primary health care and other aspects of primary prevention, such as lifestyle and behavioural changes. Each chapter will include an overview of the literature, and, possibly, some original data from European countries.

Much of the scientific evidence on access to preventive health services by migrants, as well as to primary care, is available from the USA and Australia, while the availability of information in European countries on this issue is scarce (Rosano 2017; Uiters 2009; Levecque 2012). On the other hand, the American healthcare system differs substantially from European systems in terms of the service providers as well as payers so that comparisons with European countries are challenging. For this reasons, the book is focused on the European context. The book also investigates the possible reasons for the existing inequalities among migrants and native populations.

The book is organized in nine chapters. The first chapter evaluates access to medical examination in the absence of disorders or symptoms by migrants, taking into account cultural, socioeconomic, and demographic factors. Chapters 2, 3, and 4 analyse the access to specific PHS, such as infant vaccinations, female cancer screening and colorectal screening. In chapter 5, we examine the available literature in advocacy of bridging the research and policy gap between the primary and preventive care required by and the care provided to LGBTQ+ migrants, refugees, and asylum seekers. Chapter 6 focuses on existing knowledge on health related lifestyles and intermediate health conditions, such as overweight, obesity and hypertension of migrants. Chapter 7 investigates the issue of quality of primary healthcare and preventive health services provided to migrants using hospitalization for Ambulatory Care Sensitive Conditions as a specific outcome measure. In chapter 8, we analyse the available evidence regarding adaptations of primary health for migrants. Best practices that may serve as template for those willing to implement such interventions in their primary care facility are also identified. Finally, in chapter 9, the access to PHC by migrants is discussed along with policies on migration and health, the financial crisis and PHC reforms, considering the experience of Portugal.

The book provides an exhaustive analysis of the state of the art of the access of migrants to preventive health care in the European countries, investigating the risk factors that reduce the access to PHS among migrants.

National Institute of Health   Aldo Rosano
Rome, Italy   Ornella Punzo

References

Chauvin, P., Parizot, I., & Simonnot, N. (2009). *Access to healthcare for undocumented migrants in 11 European countries*. Paris: Médecins du Monde European Observatory on Access to Healthcare.

European Commission (EC). (2008). Executive agency for health and consumers. Report on Migrant and ethnic minorities Health projects funded by European Health Programme 2003–2008, related to communicable diseases (pp. 3–4). http://ecdc.europa.eu/en/publications/Documents/090306_Health_and_Migration_projects_funded_%202003_2008.pdf

Levecque, K., Benavides, F. G., Ronda, E., & Van Ronen, R. (2012). Use of existing health information systems for migrant health research in Europe: Challenges and opportunities. In: D. Ingleby, A. Krasnik, V. Lorant, et al. (Eds.), *Health inequalities and risk factors among migrants and ethnic minorities* (pp. 53–68). Antwerp – Apeldoorn: Garant Publishers.

Liu, J., Davidson, E., Bhopal, R., White, M., Johnson, M., Netto, G., Deverill, M., & Sheikh, A. (2012). Adapting health promotion interventions to meet the needs of ethnic minority groups:

mixed-methods evidence synthesis. *Health Technology Assessment, 16*, 1–469. https://doi.org/10.3310/hta16440.

Loue, S., & Sajatovic, M. (2012). *Encyclopedia of immigrant health* (Vol. 2). New York: Springer.

MIPEX. (2017). Migrant Integration Policy Index 2015 - Health. http://www.mipex.eu/health. Accessed 6 Aug 2017.

Mladovsky, P. (2007). *Research note: Migration and health in the EU*. Brussels: European Commission.

Pace, P. (2011). The right to health of migrants in Europe. In *Migration and health in the European Union* (pp. 55–66). Maidenhead: Open University Press.

Rosano, A., Dauvrin, M., Buttigieg, S. C., Ronda, E., Tafforeau, J., & Dias, S. (2017). Migrant's access to preventive health services in five EU countries. *BMC Health Services Research, 17*(1), 588.

Uiters, E., Devillé, W., Foets, M., Spreeuwenberg, P., & Groenewegen, P. P. (2009). Differences between immigrant and non-immigrant groups in the use of primary medical care; a systematic review. *BMC Health Services Research, 9*, 76. https://doi.org/10.1186/1472-6963-9-76.

World Health Organization (WHO). (1986). Ottawa Charter for health promotion. *Canadian Journal of Public Health, 77*(6), 425–430.

Contents

Part I
Access to Preventive Health Services of Migrants and Lifestyles

Chapter 1
Access to Medical Examination for Primary Prevention Among Migrants

Anteo Di Napoli, Alessio Petrelli, Alessandra Rossi, Concetta Mirisola, and Aldo Rosano

1.1 Introduction

Migration flows from developing countries towards Europe, both for economic reasons and to flee war and persecution, have increased in the last decade, in particular towards Mediterranean countries, such as Italy, Spain and Greece (ISTAT – Geodemo 2017; Petrelli et al. 2017; Carrasco-Garrido et al. 2009; INE 2017; Galanis et al. 2013; ELSTAT 2011).

The phenomenon of immigration generated new cultural and economic challenges for each country, in particular for the health care systems (Carrasco-Garrido et al. 2009; Franchi et al. 2016). In general, migrants are healthier than native-born residents, a selection phenomenon that is known as the "healthy migrant effect", due to the selection of the subjects with better health condition can begin and face the migratory process. However, migrants represent a potentially vulnerable population, being exposed to a number of health risks before, during, and after migration (Petrelli et al. 2017; Carrasco-Garrido et al. 2009; Norredam et al. 2009).

In fact, while a number of studies have indicated that recent migrants are often healthier than their native born hosts, explaining why the demand for health care resources may be lower than that of natives, migrants' health often deteriorates with length of stay in the host country (Franchi et al. 2016). "Acculturation refers to the changes that take place among migrants due to contact with culturally dissimilar groups and influences, such as the uptake of risky health behaviors, and has been posited as an explanatory process for this deterioration" (Gazard et al. 2015).

A. Di Napoli (✉) · A. Petrelli · A. Rossi · C. Mirisola
National Institute for Health, Migration and Poverty (INMP), Rome, Italy
e-mail: dinapoli@inmp.it

A. Rosano
National Institute of Health (ISS), Rome, Italy

A. Rosano (ed.), *Access to Primary Care and Preventative Health Services of Migrants*, SpringerBriefs in Public Health, https://doi.org/10.1007/978-3-319-73630-3_1

3

Answering the health needs of migrants represents a challenge for health care services. According to the WHO the right to health implies equal and timely access to health care services, the provision of health-related education and information, and the participation of the population in health-related decisions at national and community levels. The right to health also implies equity in access to health care services for equal health needs. Health care services should be physically and financially accessible for all subgroup of the population, including vulnerable groups, and should be delivered without any discrimination. Facilities, goods, and services should respect medical ethics, being culturally and medically acceptable (UNCHR 2008; Meeuwesen et al. 2006; Devillé et al. 2011). However, some of the world's richest countries, including some of those in the European Union, have limited access to healthcare, in particular for migrants (Devillé et al. 2011; Gimeno-Feliu et al. 2016; Gimeno-Feliu et al. 2013; Diaz and Kumar 2014; Diaz et al. 2014).

Migrants do not always have access to the services they need, due to their legal status, but even in countries where access to health care is guaranteed for all migrant populations, they experience barriers for individual, socio-cultural, economic, administrative and political reasons (Devillé et al. 2011).

Structural barriers, related to legal restrictions established according to the specific health care model of each country, may limit the entitlement of the most vulnerable groups including migrants (Gil-González et al. 2015). For migrant populations, utilization of healthcare may differ from native population because of factors related to the process of migration. Particular for first-generation migrants the newcomers are less knowledgeable about the organizations of the healthcare system and how to navigate inside it (Norredam et al. 2009). Other barriers could be the limited capacity of the health services and the lack of providers meeting migrants' specific needs, hence limiting their accessibility. While entitlement relates to financing and stewardship (which mostly affects the non-universal health system model), accessibility relates to characteristics of service provision, which is more related to the National Health System model (Gil-González et al. 2015). A large body of literature has shown the risk of unequal access of migrants to health care, because migrants often face formal and informal barriers in accessing health services. A substantial variability is observed in European countries and the analyses on the issue should be conducted within the corresponding national context (Norredam et al. 2009; Gimeno-Feliu et al. 2013, 2016; Gil-González et al. 2015; Graetz et al. 2017).

Migrants may have different disease profiles from the population in host countries, and the presence of formal and informal barriers may limit their access to, and use of health services care, which may lead to social and economic deficiencies, producing greater vulnerability (Carrasco-Garrido et al. 2009; Franchi et al. 2016; Norredam et al. 2009). Formal barriers are represented by factors related to the organization of the healthcare system. They include legal restrictions on access for groups, such as undocumented migrants or asylum seekers, or those due to the cost of health care, as migrant populations in general have low socio-economic status. Organizational issues and lack of referral between services are other types of formal barriers (Norredam et al. 2009).

Socio-cultural factors, such as language, communication, and the impact with the new country may represent informal barriers to the migrants' health service utilization. On the other side, migrants, may have different expectations of health and perceptions of appropriate care, influenced by experiences with the health system in their country of origin (Cabieses et al. 2012).

Gimeno-Feliu et al. found that "barriers caused by cultural differences, language, legal status, lack of familiarity with health care provision services, employment situation and timetable incompatibility may hinder health service use, because lower levels of stable employment conditions, increase difficulty to take time off work to go to the doctor" (Gimeno-Feliu et al. 2013). Many studies found that limited language proficiency of the host country leads to inappropriate use of health services (Galanis et al. 2013; Norredam et al. 2009). Administrative complexities and lack of information play a crucial role in hindering migrants' health care access (Devillanova and Frattini 2016). Good ability to speak the language of the host country facilitates health services literacy. It has been observed that less-effective communication in relation to migrant patients may cause misunderstandings, missed appointments, non-compliance, and lead to suboptimal care and reduction of treatment adherence (Galanis et al. 2013; Norredam et al. 2009; Devillanova and Frattini 2016; van der Gaag et al. 2017).

An Italian study, based on ISTAT national survey, found that influenza vaccination coverage among all immigrants was 16.9% compared to 40.2% among Italian citizens (Fabiani et al. 2016). Differences in demographic characteristics, socio-economic conditions, and health-services utilization explain the reduced influenza vaccination coverage in most long-term immigrants compared to Italian citizens, except those from Africa and recent immigrants, suggesting the role of informal barriers (e.g., cultural and linguistic) for these sub-groups (Fabiani et al. 2016). In particular, a lower educational level has been proposed to explain the disparity in influenza vaccination among migrants, as education level is a strong predictor of preventive care receipts. Furthermore, immigrants' knowledge and attitudes towards the intervention might affect vaccination adherence (Carrasco-Garrido et al. 2009; Fabiani et al. 2016; Fiscella 2005).

Most of studies show that for a given morbidity burden, migrants' use of health services is generally lower than expected, compared to native-born populations, but other ones have found the reverse; in general the differences in the results are related to the type of health service focused by the studies (Gazard et al. 2015; Devillé et al. 2011; Gimeno-Feliu et al. 2016; Gil-González et al. 2015; Graetz et al. 2017; Glaesmer et al. 2011).

The lower use of health services could also depend on differences in attitudes and perception of health and illness, among people of different origin and culture. For example, in Spain migrants of Asian origin have much lower visit frequencies than Latin Americans, probably for their more frequent use of traditional medicines (Gimeno-Feliu et al. 2013, 2016). Furthermore it has been mentioned that migrants may have a perception of illness, they fail to use services due to fear, difficulty to take time off work, or use traditional medicines (Franchi et al. 2016; Graetz et al. 2017).

1.2   Analysis of Access to Health Care Services by Type of Setting

1.2.1   Primary Care

A Dutch study showed that general practitioners communicate differently with migrants, compared to native patients, and the consultations with migrants were shorter. Furthermore, practitioners were more verbally dominant and migrants were less demanding (Meeuwesen et al. 2006). Utilization of general practitioner services among migrants compared with natives, shows diverging rates of use in some studies and countries.

One of the reasons is that migrants are more likely to contact emergency services and less likely to visit specialist doctors or use preventive care. In fact, the utilization of accident and emergency services (bypassing general practitioner services) was higher among migrants in most studies and countries, probably because some European countries provide emergency care without any type of co-payment for the patient, making these services more affordable (Carrasco-Garrido et al. 2009; Gil-González et al. 2015; Graetz et al. 2017; Devillanova and Frattini 2016). Poor familiarity with their rights and the local health system may also influence migrants' access to care patterns. Recent migrants more frequently use emergency services, but over time they adopt natives' use patterns (Franchi et al. 2016; Norredam et al. 2009). Some authors highlighted that the overutilization of emergency services also results in higher costs when compared with accessing primary care (Graetz et al. 2017).

1.2.2   Oupatient Care

A lower utilization of outpatient specialist services by migrants compared with natives was reported by many studies (from Spain, Italy, Germany, Czech Republic), while only few studies (from Denmark, Spain, Norway) reported the opposite (Graetz et al. 2017). The migrants' general lower use of outpatient specialist services, in particular of screening services, suggest the existence of barriers in accessing these services. These barriers may be due to organizational issues, language barriers, lack of health literacy, lack of knowledge about the availability and benefits of services, and a failure to accommodate cultural differences. They could also be caused by experiences in migrants' countries of origin, where primary care and specialist services could be of poor quality, sometimes without gatekeeping systems (Norredam et al. 2009; Diaz and Kumar 2014; Diaz et al. 2014; Graetz et al. 2017; van der Gaag et al. 2017).

1.3   Use of Health Services According to Generation

Some studies observe relevant differences in health care use among first generation migrants compared to the natives and migrants' second generation. First generation migrants might be less informed about the system, while second generation, due to a higher level of acculturation, show health care utilization patterns more similar to native-born populations. In Germany, first generation migrants had a lower access to specialists and a higher frequency of visits to general practitioners (Glaesmer et al. 2011). In Spain, duration of stay was associated with higher rates of healthcare service use (Gimeno-Feliu et al. 2013, 2016). In England, recent migrants had a lower probability to be registered with a general practitioner and to use secondary health services than natives (Gazard et al. 2015). Devillanova et al. found that second-generation migrants in Italy had a lower probability of specialist visits and higher hospitalization rates (Devillanova and Frattini 2016). Franchi et al. found in Lombardy (the most peopled Italian region) an underutilization of health care between migrants even after they have been living in the region for at least 10 years (Franchi et al. 2016).

1.4   Conclusions

The lower health service use in the migrant population compared to native citizens found in many study could support the classic inverse care law described by Hart: "the availability of good medical care tends to vary inversely with the need of the population served". It is well known that people who lived on the margins of society and in disadvantaged socio-economic conditions, such as migrants, are more likely to experience poor health (Diaz and Kumar 2014; Diaz et al. 2014; Gil-González et al. 2015; Glaesmer et al. 2011).

   International evidence suggest that supply of healthcare services in universalistic systems better supports the healthcare need, but does not guarantee equity or remove the socioeconomic gradients in access and outcome (Cabieses et al. 2012). However, even in countries where access to health care is guaranteed, migrants do not always take full advantage of services available. In Spain, despite the presence of universal coverage health system offering broad legal access to migrants, the access of health-care services was lower for migrants than for natives (Gimeno-Feliu et al. 2013, 2016). A relevant issue is that universal health insurance appears to improve income equity in primary care, but not in specialist care (Glazier et al. 2009). In some European countries, like in the Netherlands and Germany (van der Gaag et al. 2017, Glaesmer et al. 2011), where a general compulsory health insurance is established and where general practitioners act, even if with a different role, as a gatekeeper between the patient and the specialist. In the Netherlands a specialist doctor cannot be approached directly by the patient, unless the patients pay an additional fee. In these cases, migrants who avoid general practitioner services might either not visit a specialist at all or try to use specialized emergency care, if provided free of charge (Schäfer et al. 2010). Thus, the differences in general practitioner gate-keeping and co-payment obligations across countries could result in different health care use of specialized care by migrants.

Moreover, according to Gimeno-Feliu et al. "health and illness are socially-construed concepts, varying greatly according to the cultural environment. Migrants may generally have a more 'utilitarian' concept of health, associated with the ability to work". Preventive activities, particularly those monitoring the evolution of chronic processes, may not be seen as priorities, as they are not acknowledged as needs, at least in their first years in the host country. As a consequence, the public health programs for preventive care should take into account the health culture of the countries of origin and their experience about health care in countries of origin that is generally characterized by major deficiencies (Gimeno-Feliu et al. 2013).

The access to healthcare of migrants is a relevant dimension of equity of care provision. To disentangle the needs of migrants' healthcare services is crucial to define effective health policy (Gimeno-Feliu et al. 2013, 2016). Appropriate policy tools to address this type of barriers are cost-effective and do not generate economically inefficient distortions on individual's behaviors (Devillanova and Frattini 2016).

Socio-economic barriers might be the main causes of disparities in access to the health care system even among second-generation migrants.

A major challenge for public health policies is integration, because the phenomenon of immigration could increase, and it is relevant to avoid problems of social cohesion (Franchi et al. 2016; Devillanova and Frattini 2016).

In conclusion, promoting migrant health care includes cultural elements from an anthropological perspective. Social and institutional changes that eliminate barriers from access to health services are fundamental in ensuring health for all (Gil-González et al. 2015).

References

Cabieses, B., Tunstall, H., Pickett, K. E., & Gideon, J. (2012). Understanding differences in access and use of healthcare between international immigrants to Chile and the Chilean-born: A repeated cross-sectional population-based study in Chile. *International Journal for Equity in Health, 11*, 68.

Carrasco-Garrido, P., Jiménez-García, R., Barrera, V. H., de Andrés, A. L., & de Miguel, A. G. (2009). Significant differences in the use of healthcare resources of native-born and foreign born in Spain. *BMC Public Health, 9*, 201.

Devillanova, C., & Frattini, T. (2016). Inequities in immigrants' access to health care services: Disentangling potential barriers. *International Journal of Manpower, 37*(7), 1191–1208.

Devillé, W., Greacen, T., Bogic, M., Dauvrin, M., Dias, S., Gaddini, A., Jensen, N. K., Karamanidou, C., Kluge, U., Mertaniemi, R., Riera, R. P., Sárváry, A., Soares, J. J., Stankunas, M., Strassmayr, C., Welbel, M., & Priebe, S. (2011). Health care for immigrants in Europe: Is there still consensus among country experts about principles of good practice? A Delphi study. *BMC Public Health, 11*, 699.

Diaz, E., & Kumar, B. N. (2014). Differential utilization of primary health care services among older immigrants and Norwegians: A register-based comparative study in Norway. *BMC Health Services Research, 14*, 623.

Diaz, E., Calderón-Larrañaga, A., Prado-Torres, A., Poblador-Plou, B., & Gimeno-Feliu, L. A. (2014). How do immigrants use primary health care services? A register-based study in Norway. *European Journal of Public Health, 25*(1), 72–78.

ELSTAT. (2011). Hellenic statistical authority. Migration 2011. http://www.statistics.gr/en/statistics/-/publication/SAM07/-. Accessed on 11 Aug 2017.

Fabiani, M., Riccardo, F., Di Napoli, A., Gargiulo, L., Declich, S., & Petrelli, A. (2016). Differences in influenza vaccination coverage between adult immigrants and Italian citizens at risk for influenza-related complications: A cross-sectional study. *PLoS One, 11*(11), e0166517. https://doi.org/10.1371/journal.pone.0166517

Fiscella, K. (2005). Commentary-anatomy of racial disparity in influenza vaccination. *Health Services Research, 40*(2), 539–549.

Franchi, C., Baviera, M., Sequi, M., Cortesi, L., Tettamanti, M., Roncaglioni, M. C., Pasina, L., Dignefa, C. D., Fortino, I., Bortolotti, A., Merlino, L., Mannucci, P. M., & Nobili, A. (2016). Comparison of health care resource utilization by immigrants versus native elderly people. *Journal of Immigrant and Minority Health, 18*, 1–7.

Galanis, P., Sourtzi, P., Bellali, T., Theodorou, M., Karamitri, I., Siskou, O., Charalambous, G., & Kaitelidou, D. (2013). Public health services knowledge and utilization among immigrants in Greece: A cross-sectional study. *BMC Health Services Research, 13*, 350.

Gazard, B., Frissa, S., Nellums, L., Hotopf, M., & Hatch, S. L. (2015). Challenges in researching migration status, health and health service use: An intersectional analysis of a South London community. *Ethnicity & Health, 20*(6), 564–593.

Gil-González, D., Carrasco-Portiño, M., Vives-Cases, C., Agudelo-Suárez, A. A., Castejón Bolea, R., & Ronda-Pérez, E. (2015). Is health a right for all? An umbrella review of the barriers to health care access faced by migrants. *Ethnicity & Health, 20*(5), 523–541.

Gimeno-Feliu, L. A., Magallón-Botaya, R., Macipe-Costa, R. M., Luzón-Oliver, L., Cañada-Millan, J. L., & Lasheras-Barrio, M. (2013). Differences in the use of primary care services between Spanish national and immigrant patients. *Journal of Immigrant and Minority Health, 15*, 584–590.

Gimeno-Feliu, L. A., Calderón-Larrañaga, A., Diaz, E., Poblador-Plou, B., Macipe-Costa, R., & Prados-Torres, A. (2016). Global healthcare use by immigrants in Spain according to morbidity burden, area of origin, and length of stay. *BMC Public Health, 16*, 450.

Glaesmer, H., Wittig, U., Braehler, E., Martin, A., Mewes, R., & Rief, W. (2011). Health care utilization among first and second generation immigrants and native-born Germans: A population-based study in Germany. *International Journal of Public Health, 56*, 541–548.

Glazier, R. H., Agha, M. M., Moineddin, R., & Sibley, L. M. (2009). Universal health insurance and equity in primary care and specialist office visits: A population-based study. *Annals of Family Medicine, 7*(5), 396–405. https://doi.org/10.1370/afm.994.

Graetz, V., Rechel, B., Groot, W., Norredam, M., & Pavlova, M. (2017). Utilization of health care services by migrants in Europe – A systematic literature review. *British Medical Bulletin, 121*, 5–18.

INE – Instituto Nacional de Estadistica. (2017). Spain 2017. http://www.ine.es/dynt3/inebase/index.htm?type=pcaxis&path=/t20/e245/p04/provi&file=pcaxis. Accessed on 10 Aug 2017.

Istat – Italian National Institute of Statistics. (2017). Geodemo: Demography in figures; Italy 2017. http://demo.istat.it/index_e.html. Accessed on 25 July 2017.

Meeuwesen, L., Harmsen, J., Bernsen, R., & Bruijnzeels, M. (2006). Do Dutch doctors communicate differently with immigrant patients than with Dutch patients? *Social Science & Medicine, 63*, 2407–2417.

Norredam, M., Nielsen, S. S., & Krasnik, A. (2009). Migrants' utilization of somatic healthcare services in Europe – a systematic review. *European Journal of Public Health, 20*(5), 555–563.

Petrelli, A., Di Napoli, A., Rossi, A., Costanzo, G., Mirisola, C., & Gargiulo, L. (2017). The variation in the health status of immigrants and Italians during the global crisis and the role of socioeconomic factors. *International Journal for Equity in Health, 16*(1), 98. https://doi.org/10.1186/s12939-017-0596-9.

Schäfer, W., Kroneman, M., Boerma, W., et al. (2010). The Netherlands health system review. *Health Systems in Transition, 12,* 1–229.

UNCHR. (2008). The right to health. Factsheet 31 OHCHR-WHO. http://www.ohchr.org/english/issues/health/right/. Accessed on 24 July 2017.

van der Gaag, M., van der Heide, I., Spreeuwenberg, P. M. M., Brabers, A. E. M., & Rademakers, J. J. D. J. M. (2017). Health literacy and primary health care use of ethnic minorities in the Netherlands. *BMC Health Services Research, 17*(1), 350. https://doi.org/10.1186/s12913-017-2276-2.

Chapter 2
Access and Barriers to Childhood Immunization Among Migrant Populations

Pier Luigi Lopalco

2.1 Vaccine Preventable Diseases in the EU: From Jenner's Vaccination to the European Vaccine Action Plan 2015–2020

Childhood vaccination programmes are considered among the most effective prevention services. In Europe vaccination programmes have a long tradition started in the late XIX century, when Jenner's vaccination was used for mass campaigns against smallpox. The modern childhood immunisation programmes have been implemented after the 1950s with the introduction of tetanus, diphtheria, polio, and subsequently pertussis vaccination. In the 1990s the introduction of hepatitis B vaccination (HBV) and, in a short time, the arrival of acellular pertussis vaccines, Haemophilus influenza type b (Hib), pneumococcal (PNC) and meningococcal (Men) conjugate vaccines improved the vaccination offer. During the latest years vaccination offer has been further enlarged with the availability of varicella, rotavirus and human papillomavirus (HPV) vaccines. Availability of new vaccines offered new opportunities but increased the complexity of the childhood vaccination programme. In many European countries introduction of new vaccines was hampered by low budget availability and competition at national level with other healthcare services (King et al. 2008). Therefore, notwithstanding the availability of safe and effective vaccines, in many EU countries there are still gaps and vaccination offer is limited to the "old" vaccines (Haverkate et al. 2012).

The EU, as well as the larger WHO European Region, adopted the European Vaccine Action Plan (EVAP) 2015–2020 (World Health Organisation 2014). Sustainability of polio-free status, elimination of measles and rubella and control of

P. L. Lopalco (✉)
Università di Pisa, Pisa, Italy
e-mail: pierluigi.lopalco@unipi.it

© The Author(s), under exclusive licence to Springer International Publishing AG, part of Springer Nature 2018
A. Rosano (ed.), *Access to Primary Care and Preventative Health Services of Migrants*, SpringerBriefs in Public Health, https://doi.org/10.1007/978-3-319-73630-3_2

hepatitis B infection are the three disease-related EVAP goals. In addition, EVAP underlines the need for having a common evidence-based approach on new vaccines introduction at European level, together with an effort to make vaccination programmes sustainable and equitably extended to all population groups.

In the EU equity is not only an issue between member states (different budget availability and subsequently different vaccination offer) but also within each country. Vaccination coverage among disadvantaged groups like migrants, refugees and travellers' communities (Roma, Sinti, Irish travellers) is often lower than the average population (Mipatrini et al. 2017).

Language barriers, lack of documents, poor education, are reported among the causes of missed opportunities for vaccination in these groups. On average, nearly 95% of children born in Europe receive the complete three-dose series of diphtheria, pertussis and tetanus vaccine by the age of 1 year. However, most of those children not accessing vaccination services belong to migrant and disadvantaged families. A strong call to "pay special attention to migrants, […], in ensuring their eligibility and access to (culturally) appropriate immunization services and information" is listed among the priority actions of the EVAP.

2.2   Poliomyelitis

The European Region was certified polio-free in 2002 and has maintained this status, notwithstanding acute threats like the outbreak in Tajikistan in 2010 (WHO 2010), the detection of silent circulation of wild polioviruses in Israel in 2013 (Shulman et al. 2014), and the cases of vaccine-derived poliovirus infection in Ukraine in 2015 (WHO 2016). Latest polio cases occurred in an EU country were reported from the Netherlands (van Wijngaarden and van Loon 1993–1994; Oostvogel PM et al. 1994). From September 1992 to February 1993, 71 polio cases and 2 deaths were confirmed in a population refusing vaccination for religious reasons. Since then no paralytic case has been reported from any EU member state in the presence of effective either acute flaccid paralysis (AFP) surveillance or environmental monitoring.

Oral polio vaccine (OPV) is the first-choice vaccine in the presence of local circulation of wild polioviruses. Once the polio-free status is certified, switch to inactivated polio vaccine (IPV) is needed in order to avoid the risk of introduction of vaccine-derived polioviruses (VDPV) in the environment. The EU countries progressively switched to IPV-only schedule starting from the polio-free status declaration. At present IPV is the only vaccine used for childhood immunisation in the EU (ECDC, Vaccine scheduler 2017). Vaccination coverage levels for three doses of IPV at 24 months are on average over 90% in most EU countries (WHO, CISID 2014). In the presence of high levels of polio vaccine coverage, the risk of having paralytic cases is very low, but the silent circulation of either wild or vaccine-derived polioviruses cannot be ruled out, as recently demonstrated in Israel. Should such silent circulation occur in an, even limited geographic area where pockets of under-vaccinated population are clustered, risk of disease becomes higher. During the recent outbreak in Ukraine, the ECDC highlighted some potential issues in countries bordering the Ukraine, like Romania, where average vaccination coverage was sub-optimal (88%). In addition, estimate on vaccine uptake in this country could have been underestimated because of lack of birth certificates or other documentation in socio-economically disadvantaged groups such as Roma. The geographical clustering of such groups can result in a situation where vaccination coverage is significantly lower than the average in the country, posing a serious threat for poliovirus circulation.

Data on polio vaccination coverage among citizens of foreign origin in EU is lacking. Few surveys have been recently carried out among refugees. In Italy, more than 99% of refugees coming from Asia and Africa and temporarily hosted in a camp were found having high immunity levels against polioviruses (Tafuri et al. 2010). In a group of refugees from Syria in Germany, 12 out of 629 (6.3%) children less than 3 years of age were positive for Sabin-like viruses in the stools, sign of recent vaccination with OPV. No wild polioviruses were found (Bottcher et al. 2015). In France, 64.4% of HIV-infected patients coming from sub-Saharian Africa had protective antibodies against the three polioviruses (Mullaert et al. 2015).

In conclusion, even if the risk for having paralytic polio cases in the EU is considered low, however children belonging to some subpopulation groups like Roma or migrants should be considered at higher risk because of low immunity levels.

2.3 Tetanus, Diphtheria, and Pertussis

Tetanus vaccination does not provide any herd immunity effect and therefore any single child not vaccinated is at high risk of disease. During the period 2010–2014, between 88 and 149 cases of tetanus have been reported in EU countries each year. The highest number of cases has been notified by Italy, Poland and France. Most of the cases occurred in adults and all fatal cases were in people aged 65 years and above (ECDC 2016d). Definitively, tetanus is under control in the EU, but still come effort must be put in place to prevent cases in those populations with low vaccination coverage or waning immunity.

Vaccination coverage among migrants have been often found to be lower in comparison with EU-born individuals. Construction workers coming from Egypt and Morocco had lower immunisation status in comparison with Italian colleagues, notwithstanding tetanus vaccination is required by Italian law for construction workers (Rapisarda et al. 2014). Workers in the agricultural sector coming from EU had higher tetanus coverage (91%) compared with non-EU workers (81%) in an Italian survey (Tabibi et al. 2013). Lower seroprevalence levels were found in the Netherlands in first-generation migrants coming from non-Western countries born before 1984, but the overall seroprevalence was over 94% in the whole population sample (Steens et al. 2010). A survey conducted in a sample of HIV infected individuals in Austria showed in migrants lower seroprevalence levels against tetanus (Grabmeier-Pfistershammer et al. 2015).

Newly arrived migrants, including children, may be a population at higher risk, due to poor access to vaccination in the country of origin. Only 27% of newly arrived migrant children in Switzerland had protective antibody levels against tetanus (de la Fuente et al. 2013).

Tetanus remains a threat for non-EU adults, especially those with higher occupational risk. In addition, special attention should be paid to the immunisation status of newly arrived migrant children.

Diphtheria cases are still reported from several EU countries. Between 2010 and 2014 number of reported cases ranged from 14 to 35 per year. In 2015, an asylum seeker originating from Afghanistan was diagnosed with respiratory diphtheria in Finland (Sane et al. 2016). He arrived in Finland from Sweden. No secondary cases were associated with this case. In France, a survey conducted among HIV-infected patients coming from sub-Saharian Africa showed protective antibodies against tetanus in 70.7% and against diphtheria in 69% of the sample (Mullaert et al. 2015).

Notwithstanding diphtheria is under control and only few clinical cases are notified in the EU, nevertheless available evidence shows that not vaccinated children are still at risk. Pertussis vaccination had a great impact on pertussis incidence worldwide. Childhood immunisation mainly aims at preventing severe pertussis cases in young infants. However, due to the limited duration of immunity after both vaccination and natural infection, repeated boosters are needed in order to decrease *Bordetella pertussis* circulation among all population groups and subsequent transmission to infants. Resurgence of pertussis is reported from several EU countries during the last years. The reasons for such phenomenon are complex and still under scientific assessment. Recently, vaccination of women during the third trimester of pregnancy is providing promising results. Very little evidence is available on vaccination coverage among migrants and disadvantaged groups for pertussis (Mipatrini et al. 2017). Any specific vaccination strategy aimed at decreasing *B. pertussis* circulation should take into consideration that migrant population may represent a disadvantaged group in terms of access to vaccination services.

2.4   Measles and Rubella

Measles and rubella are targeted for elimination in Europe. In 2016 70% and 66% of the 53 Member States in the European Region had interrupted the endemic transmission of measles and rubella, respectively (O'Connor et al. 2017). Nevertheless, large measles outbreaks as well as cases of congenital rubella still occur in many EU countries. Between January 2016 and June 2017, over 14,000 measles cases have been reported in the EU, including 35 deaths. According to the WHO Health for All database, during the decade 2004–2013, 123 new congenital rubella cases have been reported by EU countries.

A systematic review has been recently carried out in order to assess the burden of measles among migrants in the EU (Williams et al. 2016). There is little evidence available on the real incidence on measles in migrant population in Europe: those studies that mentioned migrants frequently mixed them up with indigenous religious groups or ethnic minorities. Several cases studies on measles outbreaks in Europe mention ethnic minorities or among populations at higher risk, but fail to specify whether these include recent migrants or not. The largest ethnic minority clearly related to disproportionate measles risk is the Roma/Sinti group in Bulgaria and Romania.

The latest bulletin on congenital rubella and rubella in pregnancy published by the National Institute for Health in Italy (ISS, Istituto Superiore di Sanità) reports that 25 out of 163 (15%) cases of rubella in pregnancy notified over the period 2005–2016 are in women of foreign origin (Giambi et al. 2017).

Data on vaccination coverage in migrants are not routinely collected (WHO Regional Office for Europe 2012). Few studies from individual EU countries (Germany, Italy, and Spain) report similar findings showing that migrant children are less likely to be vaccinated against measles. One German study, found that children of foreign origin had a 3-fold higher risk of being unvaccinated (Poethko-Muller et al. 2009). An Italian study reported measles vaccine coverage of 89.6% among children born outside of Italy compared with 87.3% in native children (Chiaradia et al. 2011). A study carried out in Catalonia, Spain, found a statistically significant difference in vaccine coverage rates between indigenous and immigrant children, for both the first (96.5% vs 85%) and the second dose (88.6% vs 78.3%) (Borras et al. 2007). Concerning rubella, studies carried out in Sweden and UK showed lower immunity levels in migrant than in native women (Kakoulidou et al. 2010; Hardelid et al. 2009).

In conclusion, there is strong evidence that large measles outbreaks involve ethnic minorities in the EU like Roma, but no data are routinely collected on the burden of disease among migrants. On the other hand, specific studies show that migrant children are less likely to be protected against measles in comparison with native population. In addition, disproportionate risk for rubella in pregnancy has been demonstrated in Italian women of foreign origin. In this perspective, specific measures should be implemented in order to close such potential immunization gaps and accelerate the measles and rubella elimination programme.

2.5 Meningococcal Invasive Disease

Meningococcal invasive disease is a rare but life-threatening disease in the EU. At present, the majority of cases are due to serogroup B, since serogroup C infection is mostly under control also thanks to extensive childhood vaccination programmes with meningococcal C conjugate vaccine (ECDC 2016c). Data on vaccination coverage on migrant children are not available and therefore there is no evidence of disproportionate risk of meningitis between migrant and native population (Mipatrini et al. 2017). Since risk of disease is higher in children hosted in refugee camps or living in very crowded or poor hygiene conditions, meningococcal vaccination should be considered in refugees.

2.6   Hepatitis A

EU countries present different endemicity levels for hepatitis A. According to a recent systematic review most EU countries can be considered at a very low endemicity for hepatitis A, but few counties present either low or intermediate levels that may suggest local virus circulaiton (Carrillo-Santisteve et al. 2017). Hepatitis A outbreaks still occur in Europe. Recently large multi-country outbreaks have been reported either linked to contaminated food consumption (Tavoschi et al. 2015; Scavia et al. 2017) or sexual transmission (Werber et al. 2017; Beebeejaun et al. 2017; Freidl et al. 2017). Second generation migrant children have been highlighted as peculiar risk group (Whelan et al. 2013). Second generation children are susceptible to hepatitis A having been grown in a very low endemicity country and are at high risk of infection when visiting their country of origin.

Universal childhood and adolescent hepatitis A vaccination (HAV) is effective to stop local transmission both in outbreak situations and in areas at intermediate/high endemicity (WHO 2012). In the EU universal vaccination have been implemented only in Catalonia (Spain) and Puglia (Italy). HAV is recommended to risk groups in most EU countries. Following the recent evidence, vaccination should be actively offered to second generation migrant children.

2.7   Hepatitis B

Hepatitis B virus (HBV) can cause both acute and chronic infection. Risk of chronic disease is higher if the infection is acquired during childhood. Universal children and adolescent vaccination has shown to be very effective in controlling the disease and limiting the virus spread. However, due to the presence of chronic carriers, elimination of hepatitis B is hard to achieve in a reasonable timeframe.

The prevalence of HBsAg (hepatitis B surface antigen, a marker of infection) positive individuals varies significantly across the globe, with a clear correlation between HBsAg seroprevalence and socio-economic status, with high seroprevalence level in developing countries (Schweitzer et al. 2015). Even in the EU there is a distinct geographical variation with increasing rates from West to East and from North to South (ECDC 2016b). Overall, incidence of acute hepatitis B infection is declining in the EU, probably thanks to the successful implementation of vaccination programmes. On the other hand, almost 4.5 million people live with a chronic hepatitis B virus infection in the EU (Hope et al. 2014).

Several studies have investigated the prevalence of HBV infection among migrants. A systematic assessment carried out by the ECDC reports an estimate of two million cases of chronic hepatitis B infection among migrants from intermediate/high endemic countries and a prevalence of 6% for HBsAg (ECDC 2016a, b, c, d). The ECDC study estimates that the burden of chronic hepatitis B among migrants in relation to the overall number of infected cases to be around 25%. This estimate shows that migrants are disproportionally affected by chronic hepatitis B, since the proportion of migrants in the total population is 5% for migrants coming from HBV endemic countries (ECDC 2016a). According to the ECDC assessment, migrants born in south-east or east Asian countries are among the migrant groups with the highest number of infected cases (ECDC 2016a, b, c, d). A study carried out in Amsterdam showed that the incidence of new HBV infections was higher in both first- and second-generation migrants in comparison with the Dutch-born population, showing that the risk of acquiring the infection is related to habits and living conditions of the resident migrant population, independently from the prevalence of infection in the country of origin (Whelan et al. 2012).

In Germany, both first- and second- generation children and adolescents are at higher risk of infection. In particular, children with both parents with immigration background and first-generation children are at the highest risk (Cai et al. 2011).

Studies on hepatitis B vaccine coverage among migrant children are limited. A study conducted in a rural area in Germany found similar vaccination coverage among migrant and indigenous school age population (Mikolajczyk et al. 2008).

In conclusion, acute hepatitis B infection is declining in the EU, but migrant population continue to be disproportionally at risk. In particular, knowledge on local situation is needed in order to target prevention and screening efforts towards priority migrant groups.

2.8 Barriers to Childhood Immunization Programmes Among Migrant Children

Some evidence shows that migrant children are disproportionally exposed to vaccine preventable diseases. On the other hand, data on vaccine coverage in children with migrant background are scarce because they are not routinely collected. Similarly, knowledge gaps still exist on which barriers prevent migrant groups from reaching high vaccination coverage. Lack of targeted vaccination programmes may explain this finding. Vaccination, more than other health care services, relies on robust communication strategies. In the absence of diversity-oriented and migrant-sensitive communication tools and organisation behaviour, migrant children can easily become a hard-to-reach group for vaccination programmes (Rosano et al. 2017). Recently, several countries in the EU are considering the introduction of vaccine mandates in order to counteract the increasing vaccine hesitancy among the public. A law requiring parents to vaccinate their children against 10 diseases by school age raised a vigorous debate in Italy (Day 2017). In France a similar law requiring immunisation against 11 diseases is going to be enforced starting from 2018 (APMNews 2017). Introduction of mandates may increase vaccine coverage among those migrant families that do not vaccinate their children because of lack of information or poor access to health care services. As a matter of fact, vaccine mandates for access to school may represent an effective filter to reach this population group. Finally, strong efforts should be put in place to better integrate marginalised groups like Roma/Sinti in relation to measles and rubella elimination efforts in Europe.

References

APMNews. (2017). Agnès Buzyn veut mettre en place l'obligation vaccinale pédiatrique pour 11 valences (presse). http://www.apmnews.com/nostory.php?uid=85883&objet=305244, 16 June 2017. Accessed 09 Sept 2017.

Beebeejaun, K., Degala, S., Balogun, K., et al. (2017). Outbreak of hepatitis A associated with men who have sex with men (MSM), England, July 2016 to January 2017. *Euro Surveillance, 22*(5).

Borras, E., Dominguez, A., Batalla, J., et al. (2007). Vaccination coverage in indigenous and immigrant children under 3 years of age in Catalonia (Spain). *Vaccine, 25*, 3240–3243.

Bottcher, S., Neubauer, K., Baillot, A., et al. (2015). Stool screening of Syrian refugees and asylum seekers in Germany, 2013/2014: Identification of Sabin like polioviruses. *International Journal of Medical Microbiology, 305*(7), 601–606.

Cai, W., Poethko-Muller, C., Hamouda, O., & Radun, D. (2011). Hepatitis B virus infections among children and adolescents in Germany: Migration background as a risk factor in a low seroprevalence population. *The Pediatric Infectious Disease Journal, 30*(1), 19–24.

Carrillo-Santisteve, P., Tavoschi, L., Severi, E., et al. (2017). Seroprevalence and susceptibility to hepatitis A in the European Union and European Economic Area: A systematic review. *The Lancet Infectious Diseases*. https://doi.org/10.1016/S1473-3099(17)30392-4

Chiaradia, G., Gualano, M., Di Thiene, D., et al. (2011). Health status of immigrant children: An epidemiological survey among Italian paediatricians. *Italian Journal of Public Health, 8*, 268–274.

Day, M. (2017). Doctor and MPs in Italy are assaulted after vaccination law is passed. *BMJ, 358*, j3721.

de la Fuente, I. G., Wagner, N., Siegrist, C.-A., & Posfay-Barbe, K. M. (2013). Tetanus immunity as a surrogate for past diphtheria-tetanus-pertussis immunization in migrant children. *The Pediatric Infectious Disease Journal, 32*(3), 274–277.

European Centre for Disease Prevention and Control. (2016a). Epidemiological assessment of hepatitis B and C among migrants in the EU/EEA. https://ecdc.europa.eu/sites/portal/files/media/en/publications/Publications/epidemiological-assessment-hepatitis-B-and-C-among-migrants-EU-EEA.pdf Stockholm: ECDC. Accessed 28 Aug 2017.

European Centre for Disease Prevention and Control. (2016b). Systematic review on hepatitis B and C prevalence in the EU/EEA. https://ecdc.europa.eu/sites/portal/files/media/en/publications/Publications/systematic-review-hepatitis-B-C-prevalence.pdf. Stockholm: ECDC. Accessed 28 Aug 2017.

European Centre for Disease Prevention and Control. (2016c). Annual epidemiological report 2016 – Invasive meningococcal disease. http://ecdc.europa.eu/en/healthtopics/meningococcaldisease/Pages/Annualepidemiologicalreport2016.aspx. Stockholm: ECDC. Accessed 28 Aug 2017.

European Centre for Disease Prevention and Control. (2016d). Annual epidemiological report 2016 – Tetanus. https://ecdc.europa.eu/sites/portal/files/documents/Tetanus%20AER_0.pdf. Stockholm: ECDC; 2016. Accessed 28 Aug 2017.

European Centre for Disease Prevention and Control. (2017). Vaccine scheduler. http://vaccine-schedule.ecdc.europa.eu/Pages/Scheduler.aspx. Stockholm: ECDC. Accessed 09 Sept 2017.

Freidl, G. S., Sonder, G. J., Bovee, L. P., et al. (2017). Hepatitis A outbreak among men who have sex with men (MSM) predominantly linked with the EuroPride, the Netherlands, July 2016 to February 2017. *Euro Surveillance, 22*(8).

Giambi, C., Del Manso, M., Bella, A., et al. (2017). Rosolia congenita e in gravidanza News http://www.epicentro.iss.it/problemi/rosolia/bollettino/Rosolia_congenita_news_numero%20 6%20IT.pdf. Accessed 28 Aug 2017.

Grabmeier-Pfistershammer, K., Herkner, H., Touzeau-Roemer, V., et al. (2015). Low tetanus, diphtheria and acellular pertussis (Tdap) vaccination coverage among HIV infected individuals in Austria. *Vaccine, 33*(32), 3929–3932.

Hardelid, P., Cortina-Borja, M., Williams, D., Tookey, P. A., Peckham, C. S., Cubitt, W. D., & Dezateux, C. (2009). Rubella seroprevalence in pregnant women in North Thames: Estimates based on newborn screening samples. *Journal of Medical Screening, 16*(1), 1–6.

Haverkate, M., D'Ancona, F., Giambi, C., Johansen, K., et al. (2012). Mandatory and recommended vaccination in the EU, Iceland and Norway: Results of the VENICE 2010 survey on the ways of implementing national vaccination programmes. *Euro Surveillance, 17*(22), pii=20183.

Hope, V. D., Eramova, I., Capurro, D., & Donoghoe, M. C. (2014). Prevalence and estimation of hepatitis B and C infections in the WHO European Region: A review of data focusing on the countries outside the European Union and the European Free Trade Association. *Epidemiology and Infection, 142*(2), 270–286.

Kakoulidou, M., Forsgren, M., Lewensohn-Fuchs, I., & Johansen, K. (2010). Serum levels of rubella-specific antibodies in Swedish women following three decades of vaccination programmes. *Vaccine, 28*(4), 1002–1007.

King, L. A., Lévy-Bruhl, D., O'Flanagan, D., et al. (2008). Introduction of Human Papillomavirus (HPV) vaccination into national immunisation schedules in Europe: Results of the Venice 2007 survey. *Eurosurveillance, 13*(33).

Mikolajczyk, R. T., Akmatov, M. K., Stich, H., Kramer, A., & Kretzschmar, M. (2008). Association between acculturation and childhood vaccination coverage in migrant populations: A population based study from a rural region in Bavaria, Germany. *International Journal of Public Health, 53*(4), 180–187.

Mipatrini, D., Stefanelli, P., Severoni, S., & Rezza, G. (2017). Vaccinations in migrants and refugees: A challenge for European health systems. A systematic review of current scientific evidence. *Pathogens and Global Health, 111*(2), 59–68.

Mullaert, J., Abgrall, S., Lele, N., et al. (2015). Diphtheria, tetanus, poliomyelitis, yellow fever and hepatitis B seroprevalence among HIV1-infected migrants. Results from the ANRS VIHVO vaccine sub-study. *Vaccine, 33*(38), 4938–4944.

O'Connor, P., Jankovic, D., Muscat, M., et al. (2017). Measles and rubella elimination in the WHO Region for Europe: Progress and challenges. *Clinical Microbiology and Infection: The Official Publication of the European Society of Clinical Microbiology and Infectious Diseases, 23*(8), 504–510.

Oostvogel, P. M., van Wijngaarden, J. K., van der Avoort, H. G., et al. (1994). Poliomyelitis outbreak in an unvaccinated community in The Netherlands, 1992–93. *Lancet, 344*(8923), 665–670.

Poethko-Muller, C., Ellert, U., Kuhnert, R., et al. (2009). Vaccination coverage against measles in German-born and foreign-born children and identification of unvaccinated subgroups in Germany. *Vaccine, 27*(19), 2563–2569.

Rapisarda, V., Bracci, M., Nunnari, G., et al. (2014). Tetanus immunity in construction workers in Italy. *Occupational Medicine (Oxford, England), 64*(3), 217–219.

Rosano, A., Dauvrin, M., Buttigieg, S. C., Ronda, E., Tafforeau, J., & Dias, S. (2017). Migrant's access to preventive health services in five EU countries. *BMC Health Services Research, 17*(1), 588.

Sane, J., Sorvari, T., Widerstrom, M., et al. (2016). Respiratory diphtheria in an asylum seeker from Afghanistan arriving to Finland via Sweden, December 2015. *Euro Surveillance, 21*(2).

Scavia, G., Alfonsi, V., Taffon, S., et al. (2017). A large prolonged outbreak of hepatitis A associated with consumption of frozen berries, Italy, 2013–14. *Journal of Medical Microbiology, 66*(3), 342–349.

Schweitzer, A., Horn, J., Mikolajczyk, R. T., Krause, G., & Ott, J. J. (2015). Estimations of worldwide prevalence of chronic hepatitis B virus infection: a systematic review of data published between 1965 and 2013. *Lancet (London, England), 386*(10003), 1546–1555.

Shulman, L. M., Gavrilin, E., Jorba, J., et al. (2014). Molecular epidemiology of silent introduction and sustained transmission of wild poliovirus type 1, Israel, 2013. *Euro Surveillance, 19*(7), 20709.

Steens, A., Mollema, L., Berbers, G. A. M., et al. (2010). High tetanus antitoxin antibody concentrations in the Netherlands: A seroepidemiological study. *Vaccine, 28*(49), 7803–7809.

Tabibi, R., Baccalini, R., Barassi, A., et al. (2013). Occupational exposure to zoonotic agents among agricultural workers in Lombardy Region, northern Italy. *Annals of Agricultural and Environmental Medicine, 20*(4), 676–681.

Tafuri, S., Martinelli, D., Melpignano, L., et al. (2010). High level immunity against poliomyelitis in African and Asian refugees in southern Italy. *Journal of Travel Medicine, 17*(3), 203–205.

Tavoschi, L., Severi, E., Niskanen, T., et al. (2015). Food-borne diseases associated with frozen berries consumption: A historical perspective, European Union, 1983 to 2013. *Euro Surveillance, 20*(29), 21193.

van Wijngaarden, J. K., & van Loon, A. M. (1993–1994). The polio epidemic in The Netherlands, 1992/1993. *Public Health Reviews, 21*(1–2), 107–116.

Werber, D., Michaelis, K., Hausner, M., et al. (2017). Ongoing outbreaks of hepatitis A among men who have sex with men (MSM), Berlin, November 2016 to January 2017 – linked to other German cities and European countries. *Euro Surveillance, 22*(5).

Whelan, J., Sonder, G., Heuker, J., & van den Hoek, A. (2012). Incidence of acute hepatitis B in different ethnic groups in a low-endemic country, 1992–2009: Increased risk in second generation migrants. *Vaccine, 30*(38), 5651–5655.

Whelan, J., Sonder, G., & van den Hoek, A. (2013). Declining incidence of hepatitis A in Amsterdam (The Netherlands), 1996–2011: Second generation migrants still an important risk group for virus importation. *Vaccine, 31*(14), 1806–1811.

WHO. (2016). Circulating vaccine-derived poliovirus outbreaks in 5 countries, 2014–2015. *Releve Epidemiologique Hebdomadaire, 91*(6), 71–72.

WHO Country office Tajikistan, Regional Office for Europe, & European Centre for Disease Prevention and Control. (2010). Outbreak of poliomyelitis in Tajikistan in 2010: Risk for importation and impact on polio surveillance in Europe? *Euro Surveillance, 15*(17).

Williams, G. A., Bacci, S., Shadwick, R., et al. (2016). Measles among migrants in the European Union and the European Economic Area. *Scandinavian Journal of Public Health, 44*(1), 6–13.

World Health Organisation. (2012). WHO position paper on hepatitis A vaccines – June 2012. *Releve Epidemiologique Hebdomadaire,* WHO Regional Office for Europe, Copenhagen, Denmark, *87*(28/29), 261–276.

World Health Organisation. (2014). Centralized information system for infectious diseases (CISID). WHO Regional Office for Europe, Copenhagen, Denmark, http://data.euro.who.int/cisid/?TabID=425116. Accessed 09 Sept 2017.

World Health Organization (WHO) Regional Office for Europe. (2012). Surveillance guidelines for measles, rubella and congenital rubella syndrome in the WHO European Region.

World Health Organization (WHO) Regional Office for Europe. (2014). European Vaccine Action Plan 2015–2020.

Chapter 3
Female Migrants' Attitudes and Access to Cervical and Breast Cancer Screening in Europe

Sandra C. Buttigieg and Adriana Pace

3.1 Introduction

Research has widely shown that migrant women have a universal lower participation rate in breast and cervical cancer screening programmes when compared to autochthonous women (Fontana and Bischoff 2008; Vermeer and Van den Muijsenbergh 2010; Azerkan et al. 2012; Lofters et al. 2011; Ginsburg et al. 2015; Campari et al. 2016). In addition, they also manifest lower cancer survival rates when compared to corresponding national averages (Ginsburg et al. 2017; American Cancer Society 2017).

Considering the increase in the phenomenon of migration, it is disconcerting that they are less likely to make use of screening as it has been widely reported that early detection and screening represent the best strategy for increasing survival rate (World Health Organisation 2014; European Commission 2017).

There are several reasons why policymakers and healthcare professionals should be made aware of the phenomena of ethnic and cultural diversity in the populations that health systems serve to date. The migrant population is consistently rising. For example, in 2010, the European Union (EU) hosted 31.4 million migrants, amounting to 6.3% of EU residents (Vasileva 2011). Illness may impede the integration processes of migrants in host countries as health affects their ability to engage in society in general. This may lead to further marginalization and social isolation, which again may affect health in a negative way. This is even more salient in women. The more traditional culture of the immigrant groups protects women more than men by their family (Van Ours and Veenman 2006). This infers that by and large, women integrate less within the host society, and therefore less likely to access education, health, work and other social activities. Furthermore, there is the ethical,

S. C. Buttigieg (✉) · A. Pace
University of Malta, Msida, Malta
e-mail: sandra.buttigieg@um.edu.mt

© The Author(s), under exclusive licence to Springer International Publishing AG, part of Springer Nature 2018
A. Rosano (ed.), *Access to Primary Care and Preventative Health Services of Migrants*, SpringerBriefs in Public Health, https://doi.org/10.1007/978-3-319-73630-3_3

legal as well as moral argument, which is based on the notion of "the right to the highest attainable health". This right was first described by the World Health Organisation (WHO) in 1946 and was then reiterated in other recent declarations (WHO 1978, 1998). More recently, the 2008 Resolution of the World Health Assembly on the "Health of migrants" called for a number of steps to improve migrant health, including ensuring equitable access to health services (World Health Assembly 2008). Another argument is of equity in access, which is a fundamental objective for many healthcare systems. An equitable healthcare system implies that resource allocation and access are determined by patients' need, irrespective of factors such as ethnicity or migration status (Rechel et al. 2011). Last but not least is the financial aspect as migration has a vast impact on the economy of the host country. Early detection leads to a reduction in advanced stage disease. This implies reduced costs due to less radical treatment, fewer out-patient clinic visits and a healthier working population (IARC 2002). Therefore, for these reasons health systems should better adapt to migrants' health needs and should ensure migrants' abilities to access healthcare.

Despite the emerging migrants' health problems for many European countries, we have mainly identified research originating from the United Sates (US) and Canada. For this reason, we referred to the wider literature to better understand the female migrants' attitudes and access to cervical and breast cancer screening, drawing comparisons whenever possible.

3.2 Factors Affecting Participation

There are a multitude of factors affecting breast and cervical cancer screening participation. Each of the following sections will describe the several factors, which potentially have an impact on participation of immigrant women. The first section will describe variables that are dependent on the country's policies and structure, namely entitlement and access to healthcare. In the second part, we will discuss personal variables including the socioeconomic, socio-demographic and psychosocial factors. Understanding these structural and personal factors, which hinder or facilitate breast and cervical cancer screening, is imperative as this may help to reduce the personal and societal costs of late cancer detection (Brown et al. 2006).

3.2.1 Entitlements and Access to Healthcare in Europe

Disparities in access and entitlements to healthcare exhibited by exclusionist countries can be one of the main factors leading to poor health of the immigrant population (Malmusi 2014). To our knowledge, there is no evidence directly comparing access to breast and cervical cancer screening between immigrant and native women in Europe. Most of the conducted research was carried out on the level of

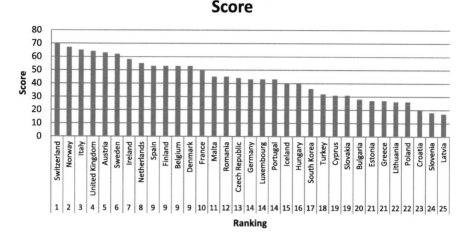

Fig. 3.1 Health Integration Policy Index of European Countries (Migration Integration Policy Index 2015)

participation rather than specifically on entitlement or access to healthcare (Fontana and Bischoff 2008; Campari et al. 2016). However, the Migrant Integration Policy Index (MIPEX 2015) compares the overall health system responsiveness to immigrants' needs by measuring four dimensions, namely entitlements, access policies, response services and mechanisms for change. As highlighted in Fig. 3.1, in Europe there are major differences, which emerge in immigrants' healthcare coverage and ability to access services between countries.

Policies are favourable in the Nordics (Norway, Sweden and Finland), English-speaking countries such as the United Kingdom, as well as countries that are major destinations for immigrants including Italy, Switzerland and Austria. Furthermore, it is evident from Fig. 3.1 that targeted migrant health policies are usually more responsive to migrant needs in countries with higher Gross Domestic Products (GDP). In addition, some of the highest ranking countries have established specific national policies aimed at improving migrant health that go beyond statutory or legal entitlements. These countries include Austria, England, France, Germany, Ireland, Italy, the Netherlands, Portugal, Spain, Sweden and Switzerland (Rechel et al. 2011).

Switzerland has ranked number one as the most responsive to immigrants' healthcare needs (MIPEX 2015). The Swiss Federal Office of Public Health (FOPH) has joined forces with the WHO and has developed a migration-specific strategy named Migration and Public Health. The main aim of this strategy was to reduce health inequalities by delivering a healthcare system that is accessible for all. This five-field intervention strategy prioritised the domains of prevention, education, research, health promotion and therapy for traumatised asylum seekers (FOPH 2002).

On the other hand, countries where numbers of migrants are very low such as in Bulgaria, Poland and Slovakia, little or nothing has been done to adapt service delivery to immigrants' needs. Austerity measures also play a major role in Greece. Other health systems that are poorly responsive or inclusive in countries with restrictive integration policies include most of Central and Southeast Europe (MIPEX 2015).

Despite the EU's declared objective to harmonise the entitlements of immigrant persons, studies demonstrate considerable, but varied, health inequalities between migrants and non-migrants (Mladovsky 2007). This problem is mostly prevalent for asylum-seekers and undocumented migrants (Karl-Trummer et al. 2010). The Council of the European Union (2003) highlighted minimum standards for asylum-seekers. These consisted of emergency care, essential treatment of illness, and necessary medical or other assistance for applicants with special needs. Nevertheless, in far too many EU member states, these minimum standards are still not met (Rechel et al. 2013).

Similar to Europe, in the US, there is inadequate access to healthcare, particularly for immigrants (Goldman et al. 2014). In addition, having health insurance is a key predictor of access to healthcare, particularly for immigrants (Siddiqi et al. 2009).

In the US there are several major public programmes, including Medicaid, which provide economic, health, and nutritional support to low-income families. Although immigrants may requires assistance through these programmes as a result of low wages and limited health insurance in comparison to nationals, they have less access to health and human services programmes. This limited access reflects stricter programme eligibility requirements, and additional barriers to access that lead eligible immigrants to take up these benefits at lower rates (Pereira et al. 2012).

Studies have shown that even if immigrant women have the same access to screening programmers when compared to resident women, participation is still lower (Ivanov et al. 2010; Campari et al. 2016; Dunn et al. 2017). This implies that migrants face other obstacles in accessing health services that go beyond legal restrictions. These obstacles include psychosocial, socioeconomic and socio-demographic factors.

3.3 Psychosocial Barriers

3.3.1 Language Barrier

Several studies document that language barrier can hinder access to healthcare, reduce the quality of care as well as result in dissatisfaction (Lim 2010; Karliner et al. 2011). Lim (2010) studied the effects of linguistic barriers on health outcomes and access in relation to cancer screening for Asian American women. It was evident that language proficiency influenced the participation rate, as English-speaking Asian American women were more likely to undergo cervical cancer screening (Lim 2010).

3.3.2 Cultural Barriers

Several studies documented cultural barriers between different immigrant groups (Ivanov et al. 2010; Lofter et al. 2011; Harcourt et al. 2014; Dunn et al. 2017). Abernethy et al. (2005) document that immigrant populations have culturally influenced attitudes and beliefs that can encourage or impede healthy behaviours such as participating in screening programmes. Examples of cultural attitudes and beliefs include fatalism, lack of perceived vulnerability, and unfamiliarity with the concept of screening (Dunn et al. 2017).

Harcourt et al. (2014) in a cross-sectional survey among African women in Minnesota reported that Somali women had higher participation rates in mammogram use while a lower rate of Pap testing when compared to other African immigrant women. In line with other studies (Cronan et al. 2008; Abdullahi et al. 2009), the author concluded that since Pap smear consists of a more invasive and personal procedure this may pose cultural barriers and may hinder these women from utilising screening services (Harcourt et al. 2014).

In previous studies, discrimination from healthcare professionals has also been shown to play a role in outcome disparities between different races as immigrant women have been prescribed different treatments. For example, Del Carmen et al. (1999) reported that black women were less likely to receive a radical hysterectomy than white women for early stage cervical cancer. Another study reported that they were less likely to receive intra-cavity radiation therapy for locally advanced disease (Mundt et al. 1998).

Another finding, which further highlights the importance of factors associated with culture, is the fact that having a family doctor who is from the same country of origin as the woman significantly increases the chances of being screened (Vahabi et al. 2016). Vahabi et al. (2016) attributed this positive relationship due to the fact that physicians from the same origin/ethnic group may overcome language barriers and have a better understanding of women's behavioural and cultural norms. Similarly, other studies have shown that the gender of healthcare professional also impacts the level of screening participation as male healthcare providers may increase the immigrants' women anxiety (Akers et al. 2007; Lofters et al. 2011).

3.3.3 Socioeconomic Barriers

Individuals with lower socioeconomic status have disproportionately higher cancer incidence rates and mortality rates than those with higher socioeconomic status, both among foreign-born women as well as among the general population. Low-income women have frequently been deemed as vulnerable to under-screening, regardless of demographic factors such as race/ethnicity (Lofters et al. 2011). In fact, women in lower socioeconomic groups often present with advanced stage disease and are less likely to receive standard regimens of treatment (Siegel et al. 2015).

Unfortunately, ethnic minorities including immigrant women disproportionately experience lower socioeconomic status (Weissman and Schneider 2005). In addition, women are at a greater risk of poverty when compared to their male counterparts (Eurostat 2017).

It is interesting to note that most of the studies which describe a low socioeconomic group as a factor affecting level of participation in cancer screening originate from the US (Weissman and Schneider 2005; Lim 2010; Siegel et al. 2015). The impact of socioeconomic factors may be much higher in the US where the Private Mixed Health Services Model applies as it is financed both privately and publicly. Privately, it is characterised by individual and employer contributions. Public systems that assist the most vulnerable patients include Medicare, Medicaid, the State Children's Health Insurance Programme and others, such as the Veterans Affairs Programme (Buttigieg et al. 2015). Public insurance is available for those 65 years of age and older, those with disabilities, and those at certain levels of the federal poverty level. Although there is public and private insurance in the US, the number of uninsured individuals continues to grow (Ivanov et al. 2010). It is evident that when compared with persons of similar socioeconomic status, uninsured and underinsured Americans receive fewer needed health services and suffer worse outcomes. Hence, lack of adequate health insurance may be one of the most important problems contributing to disparities in cancer diagnosis, treatment, and outcomes (Chatterjee et al. 2016).

3.4 Socio-Demographic Factors

3.4.1 Duration of Residence

Veermer and Van den Muijsenbergh (2010) reported that the attendance of migrant women at the national breast cancer screening in the Netherlands increased from 51% in 1997–1998 to 63% ten years after. Although in this study there were no data available about the factors associated with this increase, the authors attributed this increase to the fact that most women involved in the screening have lived for a longer period in the Netherlands. In fact the authors recommend prospective studies to get more insight on the factors contributing to higher attendance rates.

These findings are in line with other studies originating from the US as women with a longer duration of residence were more likely to screen for breast and cervical cancer (Brown et al. 2006; Harcourt et al. 2014). These differences may be due to the fact that women who have lived longer in the US are more likely to be proficient in English, and more acquainted with and have better skills at navigating the seemingly complex US health system. In addition, they are also likely to be different in respect to cultural factors, such as concerns related to modesty and cancer screening knowledge (Harcourt et al. 2014).

Vahabi et al. (2016) observed higher screening rates for immigrant women who lived longer in Canada, however, the rates never reached those of their native-born peers for many immigrant groups. These findings imply that a longer time spent in foreign country increases participation however it does not fully eliminate other socio-demographic, socioeconomic and structural barriers to screening.

3.5 Specific Immigrant Groups and Sub-groups that are Less Participative

According to Vahabi et al. (2016), studies researching breast cancer screening participation by immigrant women often consider them as a homogenous group. These studies fail to account for the diversity that exists among these subgroups. Immigrants are a heterogeneous group consisting of not only diverse ethnic, cultural, and religious affiliations, but also trajectories of acculturation that are based on the circumstances of their immigration (e.g. immigration class). These factors in turn can heavily influence immigrant women's health, health behaviours, and healthcare utilisation.

Vahabi et al. (2016) have shown that despite similarities among immigrant women regarding their low breast cancer screening utilisation, there were significant differences between subgroups living in Canada in their patterns of participation. For example, *South Asian* women had the lowest overall rate of participation while women from the Caribbean, Latin America, and Western Europe had higher screening rates.

In another study, Andreeva and Pokhrel (2013) reported that Eastern European immigrants demonstrated low health-related self-efficacy and an external locus of control as they had little health motivation while also relied on healthcare providers' initiative on screening referral. Furthermore, Easter European immigrants lacked knowledge about prevention. Regardless of the host country, healthcare access or educational level, these women largely displayed an external locus of control regarding health matters. This attitude towards health is worrying since it points to their susceptibility to cancer, as well as to other serious conditions for which personal actions and responsibilities are critical.

3.6 What Can be Done?

To ensure equity in health and healthcare for all patients, health systems need to consciously and systematically incorporate the needs of migrants into all aspects of health service planning and implementation (Forteir 2010). Towards this end, initiatives have been developed in the US and Europe aimed at building "culturally competent" or "migrant-friendly" healthcare institutions (European Migrant Friendly Hospitals Project 2004; Hudelson et al. 2014). These initiatives highlighted strategies such as facilitating access to professional interpreter services, training health-workers in cross-cultural communication, and adapting information to migrants' health literacy levels (Mladovsky et al. 2012).

Different countries use different strategies to overcome barriers and thus increase the participation of immigrant women. For example, in the 1980s, Sweden and Netherlands organised "community interpreting" systems in the health sector to overcome the language barrier. Furthermore, Sweden established the right to interpreters by law and in 2011 a telephone interpreter service, which was subsidised by the federal government, was set up for health professionals working in both the private and public sectors (Rechel et al. 2011). In Southern and Central Europe, interpreter services, if available, are often provided by "cultural mediators" (MIPEX 2015).

Another strategy to overcome the language barrier is to promote diversity amongst health professionals by recruiting staff with varied linguistic and cultural skills (Rechel et al. 2011). For example, Canada and the US have promoted the registration of students from migrant communities in medical and nursing schools (Fox 2005).

When planning and implementing strategies to increase participation, it is important to acknowledge that immigrants cannot be defined as a homogenous group as there are various subgroups (Vahabi et al. 2016). In fact, Percac-Lima et al. (2012) demonstrated that barriers to screening among Bosnian refugees and immigrants in the US could be overcome by using a culturally tailored, language-concordant navigator programme. Similarly, Shirazi et al. (2013) recommended a socially, culturally, and religiously tailored community-based health education programme for Muslim Afghan immigrants. These studies highlight the need for a holistic and culturally appropriate approach to promote cancer screening in general rather than focusing on a particular cancer (Vahabi et al. 2016).

Developing clinical and administrative structures adapted to migrant patient needs is not enough. Various studies emphasise the importance of training cultural competent healthcare professionals in order to be able to provide appropriate care to diverse patients (Weekers et al. 2009; Rechel et al. 2011; Hudelson et al. 2014). Cultural competence needs to be part of the overall skills, knowledge and attitudes of health professionals. Organisations and institutions have addressed this by providing academic courses to students and employer-sponsored training for practitioners (Hall et al. 2014).

Concurrently, professionals need to be made aware of their preconceptions. This means that healthcare providers need to adopt a humble and open-minded approach (Rechel et al. 2011). Furthermore, professionals need to understand the determinants of migrants' health and be capable to advise them about their access and entitlements (Weekers et al. 2009). An institutional culture consisting of shared values, norms and practices around the care of migrant patients must be developed for "migrant friendly" or "culturally competent" hospitals to be effective (Hudelson et al. 2014).

References

Abdullahi, A., Copping, J., Kessel, A., Luck, M., & Bonell, C. (2009). Cervical screening: Perceptions and barriers to uptake among Somali women in Camden. *Public Health, 123*(10), 680–685.

Abernethy, A. D., Magat, M. M., Houston, T. R., Arnold, H. L., Jr., Bjorck, J. P., & Gorsuch, R. L. (2005). Recruiting African American men for cancer screening studies: Applying a culturally based model. *Health Education & Behavior, 32*(4), 441–451.

Akers, A. Y., Newmann, S. J., & Smith, J. S. (2007). Factors underlying disparities in cervical cancer incidence, screening, and treatment in the United States. *Current Problems in Cancer, 31*(3), 157–181.

American Cancer Society. (2017). Cancer facts and figures. Atlanta. https://www.cancer.org/content/dam/cancer-org/research/cancer-facts-and-statistics/annual-cancer-facts-and-figures/2017/cancer-facts-and-figures-2017.pdf. Accessed 1 Aug 2017.

Andreeva, V. A., & Pokhrel, P. (2013). Breast cancer screening utilization among Eastern European immigrant women worldwide: A systematic literature review and a focus on psychosocial barriers. *Psycho-Oncology, 22*(12), 2664–2675.

Azerkan, F., Sparén, P., Sandin, S., Tillgren, P., Faxelid, E., & Zendehdel, K. (2012). Cervical screening participation and risk among Swedish-born and immigrant women in Sweden. *International Journal of Cancer, 130*(4), 937–947.

Brown, W. M., Consedine, N. S., & Magai, C. (2006). Time spent in the United States and breast cancer screening behaviors among ethnically diverse immigrant women: Evidence for acculturation? *Journal of Immigrant and Minority Health, 8*(4), 347–358.

Buttigieg, S. C., Rathert, C., & von Eiff, W. (2015). *International best practices in healthcare management*. Bingley: Emerald Books.

Campari, C., Fedato, C., Iossa, A., Petrelli, A., Zorzi, M., Anghinoni, E., Bietta, C., Brachini, A., Brezzi, S., Cogo, C., & Giordano, L. (2016). Cervical cancer screening in immigrant women in Italy: A survey on participation, cytology and histology results. *European Journal of Cancer Prevention, 25*(4), 321–328.

Chatterjee, S., Gupta, D., Caputo, T. A., & Holcomb, K. (2016). Disparities in gynaecological malignancies. *Frontiers in Oncology, 6*(36).

Council of the European Union. (2003). Laying down minimum standards for the reception of asylum seekers. Council Directive 2003/9/EC. *Official Journal of the European Union, L 31/18-L31/25.*

Cronan, T. A., Villalta, I., Gottfried, E., Vaden, Y., Ribas, M., & Conway, T. L. (2008). Predictors of mammography screening among ethnically diverse low-income women. *Journal of Womens Health, 17*(4), 527–537.

del Carmen, M. G., Montz, F. J., Bristow, R. E., Bovicelli, A., Cornelison, T., & Trimble, E. (1999). Ethnic differences in patterns of care of stage 1A1 and stage 1A2 cervical cancer: A SEER database study. *Gynecologic Oncology, 75*(1), 113–117.

Dunn, S. F., Lofters, A. K., Ginsburg, O. M., Meaney, C. A., Ahmad, F., Moravac, M. C., et al. (2017). Cervical and Breast Cancer Screening after CARES: A Community Program for Immigrant and Marginalized Women. *American Journal of Preventive Medicine, 52*(5), 589–597.

European Commission. (2017). Implementation of cancer screening in the European Union. Report on the implementation of the Council Recommendation on cancer screening, France. https://ec.europa.eu/health/sites/health/files/major_chronic_diseases/docs/2017_cancerscreening_2ndreportimplementation_en.pdf. Accessed 20 Jun 2017.

European Migrant Friendly Hospitals Project. (2004). http://www.mfh-eu.net/public/home.htm. Accessed 21 Jul 2017.

Eurostat. (2017). Gender statistics. http://ec.europa.eu/eurostat/statistics-explained/index.php/Gender_statistics. Accessed 7 Jul 2017.

Federal Office of Public Health (FOPH). (2002). Migration and public health: The confederation's strategic orientation 2002–2006, Summary, Bern. https://www.bag.admin.ch/dam/bag/en/dokumente/nat-gesundheitsstrategien/nat-programm-migration-und-gesundheit/documents-on-the-programme/migration-health-2002-2006.pdf.download.pdf/ migration-health-2002-2006.pdf. Acessed 5 Aug 2017.

Fontana, M., & Bischoff, A. (2008). Uptake of breast cancer screening measures among immigrant and Swiss women in Switzerland. *Swiss Medical Weekly, 138*(49), 752.

Fortier, A. M. (2010). Proximity by design? Affective citizenship and the management of unease. *Citizenship studies, 14*(1), 17–30.

Fox, R. C. (2005). Cultural competence and the culture of medicine. *The New England Journal of Medicine, 353*(13), 1316–1319.

Ginsburg, O. M., Fischer, H. D., Shah, B. R., Lipscombe, L., Fu, L., Anderson, G. M., & Rochon, P. A. (2015). A population-based study of ethnicity and breast cancer stage at diagnosis in Ontario. *Current Oncology, 22*(2), 97.

Ginsburg, O., Bray, F., Coleman, M. P., Vanderpuye, V., Eniu, A., Kotha, S. R., Sarker, M., Huong, T. T., Allemani, C., Dvaladze, A., & Gralow, J. (2017). The global burden of women's cancers: A grand challenge in global health. *The Lancet, 389*(10071), 847–860.

Goldman, N., Pebley, A. R., Creighton, M. J., Teruel, G. M., Rubalcava, L. N., & Chung, C. (2014). The consequences of migration to the United States for short-term changes in the health of Mexican immigrants. *Demography, 51*(4), 1159–1173.

Hall, M. B., Guidry, J. J., McKyer, E. L., Outley, C., & Ballard, D. (2014). Assessment of health disparities related academic preparation among public health department staff. *Education in Medicine Journal, 6*(3), e5–e12.

Harcourt, N., Ghebre, R. G., Whembolua, G. L., Zhang, Y., Osman, S. W., & Okuyemi, K. S. (2014). Factors associated with breast and cervical cancer screening behavior among African immigrant women in Minnesota. *Journal of Immigrant and Minority Health, 16*(3), 450–456.

Hudelson, P., Dao, M. D., Perneger, T., & Durieux-Paillard, S. (2014). A "migrant friendly hospital" initiative in Geneva, Switzerland: Evaluation of the effects on staff knowledge and practices. *PLoS One, 9*(9), e106758.

International Agency for Research on Cancer (IARC). (2002). World Health Organisation IARC Handbooks of cancer prevention, Volume 7: Breast cancer screening, Lyon. http://www.iarc.fr/en/publications/pdfs-online/prev/handbook7/Handbook7_Breast.pdf. Accessed 11 Jul 2017.

Ivanov, L. L., Hu, J., Pokhis, K., & Roth, W. (2010). Preventive health care practices of former Soviet union immigrant women in Germany and the United States. *Home Health Care Management & Practice, 22*(7), 485–491.

Karliner, L. S., Hwang, E. S., Nickleach, D., & Kaplan, C. P. (2011). Language barriers and patient-centered breast cancer care. *Patient Education and Counselling, 84*(2), 223–228.

Karl-Trummer, U., Novak-Zezula, S., & Metzler, B. (2010). Access to health care for undocumented migrants in the EU. *Eurohealth, 16*(1), 13–16.

Lim, J. W. (2010). Linguistic and ethnic disparities in breast and cervical cancer screening and health risk behaviors among Latina and Asian American women. *Journal of Womens Health, 19*(6), 1097–1107.

Lofters, A. K., Moineddin, R., Hwang, S. W., & Glazier, R. H. (2011). Predictors of low cervical cancer screening among immigrant women in Ontario, Canada. *BMC Women's Health, 11*(1), 20.

Malmusi, D. (2014). Immigrants' health and health inequality by type of integration policies in European countries. *European Journal of Public Health, 25*(2), 293–299.

Migration Integration Policy Index (MIPEX). (2015). Health. http://www.mipex.eu/health. Accessed 26 Jun 2017.

Mladovsky, P. (2007). Migration and health in the EU. European Commission, Brussels. http://citeseerx.ist.psu.edu/viewdoc/download?doi=10.1.1.473.6615&rep=rep1&type=pdf. Accessed 21 Jul 2017.

Mladovsky, P., Rechel, B., Ingleby, D., & McKee, M. (2012). Responding to diversity: An exploratory study of migrant health policies in Europe. *Health Policy, 105*(1), 1–9.

Mundt, A. J., Connell, P. P., Campbell, T., Hwang, J. H., Rotmensch, J., & Waggoner, S. (1998). Race and clinical outcome in patients with carcinoma of the uterine cervix treated with radiation therapy. *Gynecologic Oncology, 71*(2), 151–158.

Percac-Lima, S., Milosavljevic, B., Oo, S. A., Marable, D., & Bond, B. (2012). Patient navigation to improve breast cancer screening in Bosnian refugees and immigrants. *Journal of Immigrant and Minority Health, 14*(4), 727–730.

Pereira, K. M., Crosnoe, R., Fortuny, K., Pedroza, J. M., Ulvestad, K., Weiland, C., et al. (2012). Barriers to immigrants access to health and human services programs. ASPE Research Brief. http://aspe.hhs.gov/aspe/hsp/11/immigrantaccess/ barriers/rb.shtml. Accessed 31 Jul 2017.

Rechel, B., Devillé, W., Rijks, B., Petrova-Benedict, R., & McKee, M. (2011). *Migration and health in the European Union*. Maidenhead: Open University Press. http://www.euro.who.int/__data/assets/pdf_file/0019/161560/e96458.pdf. Accessed 29 May 2017

Rechel, B., Mladovsky, P., Ingleby, D., Mackenbach, J. P., & McKee, M. (2013). Migration and health in an increasingly diverse Europe. *The Lancet, 381*(9873), 1235–1245.

Shirazi, M., Bloom, J., Shirazi, A., & Popal, R. (2013). Afghan immigrant women's knowledge and behaviors around breast cancer screening. *Psycho-Oncology, 22*(8), 1705–1717.

Siddiqi, A., Zuberi, D., & Nguyen, Q. C. (2009). The role of health insurance in explaining immigrant versus non-immigrant disparities in access to health care: Comparing the United States to Canada. *Social Science & Medicine, 69*(10), 1452–1459.

Siegel, R. L., Miller, K. D., & Jemal, A. (2015). Cancer statistics, 2015. *CA: A Cancer Journal for Clinicians, 65*(1), 5–29.

Vahabi, M., Lofters, A., Kumar, M., & Glazier, R. H. (2016). Breast cancer screening disparities among immigrant women by world region of origin: A population-based study in Ontario, Canada. *Cancer Medicine, 5*(7), 1670–1686.

Van Ours, J. C., & Veenman, J. (2006). Age at immigration and educational attainment of young immigrants. *Economics Letters, 90*(3), 310–316.

Vasileva, K. (2011). 6.5% of the EU population are foreigners and 9.4% are born abroad. *Statistics in Focus* 34/2011. Luxemburg: Eurostat.

Vermeer, B., & Van den Muijsenbergh, M. E. (2010). The attendance of migrant women at the national breast cancer screening in the Netherlands 1997–2008. *European Journal of Cancer Prevention, 19*(3), 195–198.

Weekers, J., Acuña, D. L., Sánchez, M. T. G., Pulido, S. P., Aitken, R. L. K., Benedict, R. P., & Peiro, M. J. (2009). Developing a Public health workforce to address migrant health needs in Europe. Background paper. International Organization for Migration (IOM), Brussels. http://www.migrant-health-europe.org/files/Capacity%20Building%20in%20Healthcare_Background%20Paper(1).pdf. Accessed 24 Jul 2017.

Weissman, J. S., & Schneider, E. C. (2005). Social disparities in cancer: Lessons from a multidisciplinary workshop. *Cancer Causes & Control, 16*(1), 71–74.

World Health Assembly. (2008). Health of migrants, resolution of the 61st world health assembly. World Health Organization, Geneva. http://apps.who.int/gb/ebwha/pdf_files/ WHA61-REC1/A61_REC1-en.pdf. Accessed 20 Jul 2017.

World Health Organization. (2014). Comprehensive Cervical Cancer Control A guide to essential practice. Second edition. Geneva, Switzerland. http://apps.who.int/iris/bitstream/10665/144785/1/9789241548953_eng.pdf. Accessed 12 Aug 2017.

World Health Organisation. (1946). WHO Constitution, Geneva.

World Health Organisation. (1978). The Alma Ata declaration. World Health Organization, Geneva. http://www.who.int/publications/almaata_declaration_en.pdf. Accessed 20 Jul 2017.

World Health Organisation. (1998). World health declaration, World Health Organization, Geneva. http://www.who.int/whr/1998/en/whr98_en.pdf. Accessed 20 Jul 2017.

Chapter 4
Access to Colon Cancer Screening of Migrants in Four European Countries

Ornella Punzo and Aldo Rosano

4.1 Background

Risk prevention and mitigation play a major role in reducing the incidence of cancer cases. If the exposure to cancer cannot be avoided, the next step would be making efforts to minimise the negative effects of exposure, e.g. enabling early detection of cancer cases. These strategies can be organized at an individual or at a population level. One of the main interventions at population level to decrease premature deaths is to ensure access to screening and early detection services. This type of screening can reduce dramatically the mortality from breast, cervical and colorectal cancer. Estimates show that a total of 256,670 men and women died of these three cancers in 2012 in the EU Member States (including Croatia), even though many of these early deaths were preventable (International Agency for Research on Cancer 2017). Population-based colorectal cancer screening has proven to be effective in reducing colorectal cancer incidence and mortality. The uptake of population-based programmes proved higher than spontaneous screening, confirming this type as more effective than other types of screening, such as spontaneous screening (Ferroni et al. 2012). Both letter-based and GP-based invitation programmes seemed effective, but the former appeared more cost-effective (Ferroni et al. 2012).

Therefore, the implementation of such population-based screening approaches with well-defined target population, screening intervals and appropriate follow-up would reduce the burden of these cancers in the European region. Access to quality screening services plays a major role in the success of screening programmes (International Agency for Research on Cancer 2017; European Commission 2017).

O. Punzo · A. Rosano (✉)
National Institute of Health, Rome, Italy
e-mail: aldo.rosano@iss.it

A. Rosano (ed.), *Access to Primary Care and Preventative Health Services of Migrants*, SpringerBriefs in Public Health, https://doi.org/10.1007/978-3-319-73630-3_4

Colorectal cancer (CRC) is much more common in developed countries and is associated with dietary habits and environmental risk factors. It is recommended that screening starts at around the age of 50 using faecal occult blood tests and endoscopic exams. Colorectal cancer is the second most common cancer in Europe, causing over 200,000 deaths per year (European Colorectal Cancer Screening Guidelines Working Group, 2013).

CRC screening tests are ranked in three tiers based on performance features, costs, and practical considerations. The first-tier tests are colonoscopy every 10 years and annual faecal immunochemical test (FIT). These tests are recommended regardless of being included or not in a population based type of screening, and they are also tests of choice when several alternatives are available. FIT should be offered to patients who decline colonoscopy, in a sequential fashion. FIT screening is also appropriate in populations with an estimated low prevalence of advanced neoplasia, whereas colonoscopy screening is recommended in high prevalence populations. The second-tier tests include CT colonography every 5 years, the FIT-faecal DNA test every 3 years, and flexible sigmoidoscopy every 5–10 years. A third-tier test is capsule colonoscopy every 5 years. Screening should begin at age 50 years in average-risk persons (Rex et al. 2017). CRC incidence is rising in persons under age 50, and thorough diagnostic evaluation of young persons with suspected colorectal bleeding is recommended (Rex et al. 2017).

In Europe to date, only the faecal occult blood test (FOBT) for men and women aged 50–74 years has been recommended by the EU for CRC screening (European Colorectal Cancer Screening Guidelines Working Group, 2013). Moreover, any other screening technique included should follow the principle listed by the Council of Europe Recommendation and be evidence-based. Although the use of endoscopic screening methods is increasing, the majority of colorectal cancer screening examinations performed in the EU use the evidence-based test recommended by the Council of Europe.

The current status of colorectal cancer screening in Europe shows 23 countries having their programmes either already implemented or in the planning phase, with the implementation started only in the 2000s. More than 110 million women and men are being targeted by these population-based programmes. For colorectal cancer the International Agency for Research on Cancer (IARC) and the European Commission report that there are currently population based screening programmes at national level in 15 Member States, while in 4 Member States population based screening programmes exist only in some regions, and in 9 Member States no programmes exist for the moment (but in 6 of them several CRC screening actions are scheduled for 2016) (European Commission 2017). Though a majority of the screening is still based on FOBT, large proportions of the target population have access to screening using endoscopy (flexible sigmoidoscopy or total colonoscopy). In Europe the screening interval for gFOBT/FIT programmes is 2 years in all the countries except Austria and Latvia where screening is done yearly. Within the non-population-based programmes, screening with colonoscopy is offered at 10 years interval in Austria, Czech Republic and Germany and at 5 years interval in Greece. Within population-based programmes, colonoscopy is offered once in a lifetime in

Poland as it is the case for sigmoidoscopy in Italy and England (International Agency for Research on Cancer 2017; European Commission 2017).

Eurostat shows that the self-reported screening, i.e. the proportion of people aged 50–74 years having had a colorectal cancer screening test within the specified time periods, in 2014 or nearest year, varies greatly in different European countries (European Commission n.d.). The EU-28 estimate average of the European population having had a colonoscopy ever is less than 50%. Countries such as Romania, Cyprus, Bulgaria and Estonia (followed closely by Norway) are the ones reporting the highest proportion of people who never had a colonoscopy in their life. Germany, Austria, Slovenia and Czech Republic were the countries where the above mentioned proportion was the lowest.

Secondary cancer prevention programs are particularly important for migrants because they often underuse preventive care or fail to make return medical visits, and often lack cancer awareness. Migrants are more likely to receive a diagnosis of cancer at an advanced stage. Limited access to screening is one possible reason for this. Another element to consider is that the inclusiveness of the target population database chosen to issue invitations for screening purposes depends on how complete is the database and on the eligibility of individuals, e.g. electoral registers might not include eligible foreigners or dates of birth (European Colorectal Cancer Screening Guidelines Working Group, 2013).

In the USA, colorectal screening tends to be lower for migrants than for the native population. However, screening patterns converge towards that of the native population as the length of stay in the country increases (Arnold and Razum 2012). Risk factors change over time upon arrival in the host country, and changes in a lifespan can be mixed, both positive and negative. Factors such as dietary changes, physical inactivity, weight gain and obesity, smoking, all contribute to a shift in migrant population's risk profile. Therefore, despite the presence of the well-known "healthy migrant effect", for which immigrants have a better health profile and overall lower mortality than hosts in Western countries, the convergence of mortality for hosts and immigrants with increasing duration of residence suggests that "healthy migrant effect", and negative acculturation effects may counteract each other. The "healthy migrant effect" explains how on average migrants arriving in a host country are healthy, and this is explained as they would represent a pre-selected healthier cluster of their population of origin. On the contrary, the assimilation of cultural traits of the local population, such as alcohol consumption or increased dietary fat, would lead to a deterioration of the originally better migrant health profile. Arnold et al. (2009) analysed the literature for cancer risk diversity in non-western immigrants to Europe and found that they show an overall lower all-cancer morbidity and mortality compared with the native population. Nevertheless, they noticed considerable site-specific risk diversity. While migrants from non-western countries were more prone to infections-related cancers, e.g. liver, cervical and stomach cancer, at the same time they were less likely to get cancers related to western lifestyle, e.g. colorectal, breast and prostate cancer. Therefore, there is a strong need of culturally sensitive cancer prevention and screening programmes that take into account the specific needs and risk profiles of migrants, also at the individual level.

This chapter aims at investigating the access to colorectal screening programs among migrants through a review of the literature and at analysing some original data from four European countries.

4.2   Review of the Literature

We reviewed the literature searching for original papers and reviews focusing on the uptake and the barriers to access CRC screening for migrants in Europe; in addition, we analysed original data from four European countries coming from the European Health Interview Surveys (EHIS).

The literature search was performed on Pubmed electronic database, through free Google and Google scholar search and snowballing selected articles references. The Italian grey literature was retrieved from national and regional websites, including the Ministry of Health website. The European Commission and the International Agency for Research on Cancer (IARC) websites were searched for the European grey literature. Guidelines and reports were also found in official European Union or European Commission websites.

Pubmed Search Terms
1. "migrant"[Title/Abstract] AND ("neoplasms"[MeSH Terms] OR "neoplasms"[All Fields] OR "cancer"[All Fields]) AND ("2007/09/01"[PDAT]: "2017/09/01"[PDAT]) AND "humans"[MeSH Terms].
2. "migrant"[Title/Abstract] AND "cancer screening"[Title/Abstract] AND ("2007/09/14"[PDat]: "2017/09/13"[PDat] AND "humans"[MeSH Terms]).

There are very few literature reviews regarding the access to health services in general and even less specifically focused on access to screening by migrants. The screening methods used in the original data were gFOBT (guaiac-based faecal occult blood test) and colonoscopy, while in the original articles we found FOBT, sigmoidoscopy and colonoscopy in the US (Idowu 2016), FIT (faecal immunochemical test) in the Netherlands (with colonoscopy offered to those with a positive sample) (Woudstra et al. 2016), FOBT in the UK (Robb et al. 2008), FOBT for France (Le Retraite et al. 2010). We will analyse the results comprehensively, despite that different countries have different CRC screening techniques in their programmes.

In the systematic review by Norredam et al., there are only four studies focused on screening services, and none of them refers to colorectal cancer screening; they are focused instead on mammography (2) and on cervical screening (2) (Norredam et al. 2010). Nevertheless, the findings show a lower uptake of cancer screening services among migrants compared with the indigenous population in all four studies. The systematic literature review by Graetz et al. on utilization of health care services by migrants (Graetz et al. 2017) found that all screening practices (mammography for breast cancer, cervical cytology for cervical cancer, abdominal aortic screening for aneurysm, and finally colorectal cancer screening through gFOBT or flexible sigmoidoscopy) were far less utilized by migrants than by the resident population. The studies were conducted in different European countries, such as Spain, Sweden, Germany, Denmark, Greece and the Netherlands, the only exception being a single German study involving Turkish immigrants, that showed higher screening services utilization compared to the local population (though study results were regarded as inconsistent with the European trend).

Frederiksen et al. report that participation in colorectal cancer screening was almost half as frequent in migrants compared with native Danes (Frederiksen et al. 2010). Accordingly to this study, that analysed how the participation to systematic CRC screening was affected by socioeconomic factors, low SEP (socioeconomic position) was associated with lower testing with FOBT. Moreover, non-western immigrants were also less likely to uptake the screening, but this difference was likely attributed to the lower SEP in the ethnic groups considered.

In another paper included in this systematic review by Carrasco-Garrido et al., a study was conducted on awareness and uptake of cancer screening in Spain (Carrasco-Garrido et al. 2014). By 2010, six Spanish autonomous regions had implemented population-based screening programmes for CRC, representing 40% of the total Spanish population (Ascunce et al. 2010).These programmes include men and women aged 50–69 years as their target population using faecal occult blood test (FOBT) every 2 years. Adherence to these programmes ranged from 5.4 to 21.6%. Among the results, the study shows that subjects born in Spain reported higher awareness of all cancer screening programmes and specifically of FOBT (OR 1.41; 95% CI: 1.16–1.71) than immigrants. The highest uptake was found for mammography (74.46%; 95% CI: 71.96–76.14), followed by Pap smears (65.57%; 95% CI: 63.09–66.83), PSA (Prostate-Specific Antigen) (35.19%; 95% CI: 32.43–37.94) and FOBT (9.40%; 95% CI: 7.84–11.23). However, it has to be considered that the uptake for CRC screening in Spain is overall much lower than in other European countries such as UK or Italy (e.g. 56.8% in the UK and 44.6% in Italy) (Carrasco-Garrido et al. 2014) .

The possible explanations given for the lower screening uptake among migrants range from lack of information to lack of screening tests tailored for migrants, low socio-economic status, socio-demographic or linguistic issues and finally lack of health insurance (Graetz et al. 2017). Socio-economic status, including education, employment and income, plays a significant role in migrant health in general, and since migrant populations are usually more financially disadvantaged, their health profile tends to get worse upon years after arriving in the host country (Dinesen 2011).

A paper authored by Le Retraite et al. (2010) focuses on the impact of the place of residence on participation, or lack thereof, in a CRC screening in Marseille, France. The study finds that migrant participation in CRC screening is lower compared to the non-migrant population, with differences in participation related to higher presence of migrants in a district. However, the differences observed do not seem to be attributable to migrant status, this being more likely to represent a proxy of other intrinsically related socioeconomic factors (Le Retraite et al. 2010). Another qualitative study conducted in the Netherlands (Woudstra et al. 2016) shows how a low level of Dutch language was the biggest barrier to CRC screening. Mistrust, misconceptions and low self-efficacy were all counted as other reasons for low CRC uptake. Practice implications included a request for more easily accessible information, such as verbal and visual information in the mother tongue of the recipients. A bigger involvement of the GP was also suggested as a means of higher self-efficacy. A further research paper looks at attitudes to CRC screening among minority groups in the UK (Robb et al. 2008). As also previous literature highlighted, that socioeconomic status affected CRC uptake more significantly than ethnicity alone. Regarding possible barriers to accessing CRC screening, shame and embarrassment seem to be the leading causes for disinterest towards screening programmes and lower CRC screening uptake.

A further review of the literature was performed in order to find other sources treating this subject, but it only retrieved a few articles. We performed a broader search using less and more undefined terms on Pubmed and Google, but only retrieved papers useful for describing the context.

4.3   Original Data Analysis on CRC Screening

We tried to integrate the literature available on migrants' access to CRC screening through the analysis of data coming from European Health Interview Surveys (EHISs) and National Health Interview Surveys (HIS) and other data sources from different European countries on colorectal screening coverage. The screening methods considered are gFOBT and colonoscopy, which are among the techniques recommended by the American and European CRC screening guidelines (Rex et al. 2017; von Karsa et al. 2012).

The data sources were the HISs, respectively 2011 for Spain, 2012–2013 for Italy, 2013 for Belgium and 2014 for Portugal. The indicator chosen was the percentage of persons (aged 50–74) reporting a colorectal cancer screening in the past 3 years. The proportion of interviewed subjects reporting a gFOBT colorectal cancer screening was 17.2% (17.5% among nationals and 11.1 among migrants) (Table 4.1).

Information about colonoscopy was analysed for Italy only. Those who underwent a colonoscopy in the last 5 years, aging 50–74 years, were 13.1% among nationals and 7.5% among migrants. Those who never underwent a colonoscopy were 83.4% among nationals and 91.2% among migrants.

4.4   Discussion

Early detection during screening programs for colorectal cancer is a key factor for better survival in high-risk groups. In the original data, focus of this analysis, the proportion of interviewed subjects reporting a colorectal cancer screening was very

Table 4.1 Percentage of subjects who reported a gFOBT by country and immigrant status in four EU countries. Age 50–74

	Belgium	Italy	Portugal	Spain	Total
Nationals					
In the year	8.7	2.5	17.8	4.0	5.0
1–2 year	7.8	10.0	9.5	2.3	8.9
2–3 year	4.1	4.8		1.0	3.6
>3 or never	79.4	82.7	72.7	92.7	82.5
Migrants					
In the year	10.9	1.7	14.3	3.5	4.0
1–2 year	7.1	5.1	3.8	2.5	4.8
2–3 year	6.0	2.2		1.6	2.3
>3 or never	76.0	91.0	81.9	92.4	88.9

low (1 out of 7). Among the considered countries, in Italy, Portugal and Spain the proportion of migrants who reported CRC screening was much lower that of nationals. In other countries, such as the UK, this appears to be due to a general lack of information about colorectal cancer, which was more pronounced among some minority groups (Robb et al. 2008).

Cultural factors may also play a role, e.g. fatalism (the perception of everything as being ordained by fate) was found to be associated with a lower uptake of colorectal cancer screening among elderly African Americans compared to elderly white participants in the USA (Powe 1995). Several studies highlighted how being foreign-born correlates with a lower CRC screening uptake. This may be due to a lack or lower availability of organized CRC screening in the country of origin. Lower awareness of CRC screening is also thought to be associated to lower access to healthcare services in settings such as the USA, where access to public healthcare and health coverage is not guaranteed to the whole population and the non-universalistic health system is quite different from how it is organized in Europe (Idowu 2016). Therefore, the need of wider health education and information provision for immigrants are listed as possible solutions. Moreover, a lack of knowledge of colorectal cancer family history may translate into a low perceived risk of CRC. The health belief model substantially predicts these results. This model theorized that people's beliefs about susceptibility to disease, and about their perceptions of the benefits of prevention, influenced their readiness to act (Idowu 2016).

In the USA, although screening uptake is raising for both immigrant and non immigrant groups, gaps still remain and are linked to citizenship and insurance status (Reyes and Miranda 2015). Wide variations in the recommendations given by the GPs were also noted, suggesting that the first step to improve screening uptake among ethnic minorities could be ensuring that GPs recommend guideline-aligned screening to all patients. Also relevant is using computerized medical records, which through reminders increased the screening uptake, while minimizing the health inequalities among the migrant population (Reyes and Miranda 2015).

Although medical issues and guidelines are defined and meant to be internationally acceptable in principle and application, the context in which patient needs are defined and expectations met, remain one of the biggest challenges. One of the key solutions would lie in recognizing individual needs and resources in order to deal appropriately with increasing cultural and ethnic diversity in the context of a society whose priorities are currently heavily dictated by profit, efficiency, tighter regulations and standardized practices (Norredam et al. 2006).

4.5   Conclusions

Many factors may contribute to hindering migrant access to preventive health services (PHSs), such as length of stay in the host country, ethnic background, culture, religion, levels of health literacy and integration, resulting in inequitable access of migrants to CRC screening. Social factors have a significant role in migrant health and the direction of the causal processes is not always clear. Barriers to access non-urgent health services are identified as organizational issues (both on the administration and on the physician sides), language barriers (and lack of interpreters, which for example prevents from performing telephone consultations), lack of health literacy (not recognizing symptoms and potentially life-threatening health risks), lack of knowledge about availability and benefits of the services, failure in offering culture-sensitive options (Graetz et al. 2017). It is well known that one of the main barriers for screening uptake in the USA is represented by the insurance status (Reyes and Hardy 2015), but it may come a bit as a surprise that the situation is similar in Canada too (Gesink et al. 2014). In Europe, entitlements for migrants vary from country to country (Huddleston 2015).

There is urgent need for a deeper understanding of the barriers between migrants and CRC screening uptake as well as for more and better longitudinal studies, mixed methods and intervention studies in order to obtain better indicators of social determinants and integration. Moreover these indicators also need to be significant at an international level. Many researchers argue that there is urgent need of "intersectional, integrated, multivariate and multilevel approaches" (Ingleby 2012).

Public health issues, such as access to health services and screening, are intrinsically related to poverty, and poverty to immigration, especially in countries where immigrants are not granted free access to preventive care or where health services are not enough culturally sensitive. A so-called intersectional approach would take into account how the multifaceted issues and obstacles to access CRC screening can be tackled, how these barriers interact with each other, how different research and operational areas of action intersect and how this intersection can be utilised to better understand how to guarantee the access to CRC screening to migrants.

Intersectionality, a term coined by Kimberlé Williams Crenshaw, recognizes that certain individuals face multiple and intersecting forms of structural discrimination.

On this issue Östlin (2011) asks: "What are the interactions between the axes of social differentiation and how do these contribute to the patterning of inequity at population level? More specifically, how do economic status, ethnicity, and gender intersect to shape health risks and outcomes?" (Östlin 2011). In order to tackle inequities in health we need an integrated approach that looks at different factors that contribute to create them at the same time. This approach would harmonize the traditional conflicting research fields of social determinants of health and ethnicity studies (Ingleby 2012).

In reality, only a few prevention programmes exclusively target migrant groups (Mackenbach et al. 2008). Preventive health services should be responsive to patient diversity, probably more than other health services. There is a need for diversity-oriented, migrant-sensitive prevention and a need for prevention programs addressing migrants that are large-scale, evidence-based, sustainable and regularly evaluated. Policies oriented to removing impediments to migrants' access to preventive interventions are crucial, in order to encourage more positive actions for those facing the risk of intersectional discrimination (Rosano et al. 2017). An intersectional approach, in the case of CRC screening, would therefore take into account different aspects of the barriers and issues relevant to migrants' access to screening. This would be made possible by enquiring the lives, thoughts, ideas of the group under study. Culture-sensitive services, tailored to the specific needs and expectations of specific ethnic subgroups would be the major step on this path.

References

Arnold, M., & Razum, O. (2012). Cancer prevention. In S. Loue, M. Sajatovic (Eds.), *Encyclopedia of immigrant health*, (pp. 354–356). KissLibrary. Springer, New York. https://doi.org/10.1007/978-1-4419-5659-0_116.

Arnold, D., Girling, A., Stevens, A., & Lilford, R. I. (2009). Comparison of direct and indirect methods of estimating health state utilities for resource allocation: Review and empirical analysis. *BMJ, 339*, 2688.

Ascunce, N., Salas, D., Zubizarreta, R., Almazán, R., Ibáñez, J., & Ederra, M. (2010). Cancer screening in Spain. *Annals of Oncology, 21*(Supplement 3), 43–51.

Carrasco-Garrido, P., Hernandez-Barrera, V., Lopez de Andres, A., Jimenez-Trujillo, I., Gallardo Pino, C., & Jimenez-Garcia, R. (2014). Awareness and uptake of colorectal, breast, cervical and prostate cancer screening tests in Spain. *European Journal of Public Health, 24*, 264–270.

Dinesen, C. (2011). Inequality in self-rated health among immigrants, their descendants and ethnic Danes: Examining the role of socioeconomic position. *International Journal of Public Health, 56*, 503–514.

European Colorectal Cancer Screening Guidelines Working Group, E.C.C.S.G.W, et al. (2013). European guidelines for quality assurance in colorectal cancer screening and diagnosis: Overview and introduction to the full supplement publication. *Endoscopy, 45*, 51–59.

European Commission. (2017). Commission Implementing Decision of 26.1.2017 concerning the work programme for 2017 in the framework of the third Programme of the Union's action in the field of health (2014–2020) and the EU financial contribution to the WHO Framework Convention on Toba.

European Commission. (n.d.). Eurostat – Database. Brussels. Available at: http://ec.europa.eu/eurostat/data/database. Accessed 1 Aug Brussels, 2017.

Ferroni, E., Camilloni, L., Jimenez, B., Furnari, G., Borgia, P., Guasticchi, G., & Giorgi Rossi, P. (2012). How to increase uptake in oncologic screening: A systematic review of studies comparing population-based screening programs and spontaneous access. *Preventive Medicine, 55*, 587–596.

Frederiksen, B. L., Jørgensen, T., Brasso, K., Holten, I., & Osler, M. (2010). Socioeconomic position and participation in colorectal cancer screening. *British Journal of Cancer, 103*, 1496–1501.

Gesink, D., Mihic, A., Antal, J., Filsinger, B., Racey, C. S., Perez, D. F., Norwood, T., Ahmad, F., Kreiger, N., & Ritvo, P. (2014). Who are the under- and never- screened for cancer in Ontario: A qualitative investigation. *BMC Public Health, 14,* 495.

Graetz, V., Rechel, B., Groot, W., Norredam, M., & Pavlova, M. (2017). Utilization of health care services by migrants in Europe—a systematic literature review. *British Medical Bulletin, 121,* 5–18.

Huddleston, T. (2015). Migrant integration policy index. Available at: http://www.mipex.eu/. Accessed 1 Sept 2017.

Idowu, K. A. (2016). Place of birth, cancer beliefs and being current with colon cancer screening among US adults. *Annals of Gastroenterology, 29,* 336–340.

Ingleby, D. (2012). Ethnicity, migration and the "social determinants of health" agenda*. *Psychosocial Intervention, 21,* 331–341.

International Agency for Research on Cancer (IARC). (2017). Cancer Screening in the European Union Report on the implementation of the Council Recommendation on cancer screening. Brussels: European Commission.

Le Retraite, L., Eisinger, F., Loundou, A., & Auquier, P. (2010). Sociogeographical factors associated with participation in colorectal cancer screening. *Gastroentérologie Clinique et Biologique, 34,* 534–540.

Mackenbach, J. P., Stirbu, I., Roskam, A. J., Schaap, M. M., Menvielle, G., Leinsalu, M., Kunst, A. E., & European Union Working Group on Socioeconomic Inequalities in Health. (2008). Socioeconomic inequalities in health in 22 European countries. *New England Journal of Medicine, 358,* 2468–2481.

Norredam, M., Mygind, A., & Krasnik, A. (2006). Access to health care for asylum seekers in the European Union--a comparative study of country policies. *European Journal of Public Health, 16,* 286–290.

Norredam, M., Nielsen Smith, S., & Krasnik, A. (2010). Migrants' utilization of somatic health-care services in Europe-a systematic review. *European Journal of Public Health, 20,* 555–563.

Östlin, P. (2011). Priorities for research on equity and health: Towards an equity-focused health research agenda. *PLoS Medicine, 8,* e1001115.

Powe, B. D. (1995). Fatalism among elderly African Americans. Effects on colorectal cancer screening. *Cancer Nursing, 18,* 385–392.

Rex, D. K., Boland, C. R., Dominitz, J. A., Giardiello, F. M., Johnson, D. A., Kaltenbach, T., Levin, T. R., Lieberman, D., & Robertson, D. J. (2017). Colorectal cancer screening: Recommendations for physicians and patients from the U.S. Multi-Society Task Force on Colorectal Cancer. *American Journal of Gastroenterology, 153,* 307–323.

Reyes, A. M., & Hardy, M. (2015). Health insurance instability among older immigrants: Region of origin disparities in coverage. *The Journals of Gerontology Series B: Psychological Sciences and Social Sciences, 70,* 303–313.

Reyes, A. M., & Miranda, P. Y. (2015). Trends in cancer screening by citizenship and health insurance, 2000–2010. *Journal of Immigrant and Minority Health, 17,* 644–651.

Robb, K. A., Solarin, I., Power, E., Atkin, W., & Wardle, J. (2008). Attitudes to colorectal cancer screening among ethnic minority groups in the UK. *BMC Public Health, 8,* 34.

Rosano, A., Dauvrin, M., Buttigieg, S. C., Ronda, E., Tafforeau, J., & Dias, S. (2017). Migrant's access to preventive health services in five EU countries. *BMC Health Services Research, 17,* 588.

von Karsa, L., Patnick, J., & Segnan, N. (2012). European guidelines for quality assurance in colorectal cancer screening and diagnosis. First Edition – Executive summary. *Endoscopy, 44*(S 03), SE1–SE8.

Woudstra, A. J., Dekker, E., Essink-Bot, M. L., & Suurmond, J. (2016). Knowledge, attitudes and beliefs regarding colorectal cancer screening among ethnic minority groups in the Netherlands – a qualitative study. *Health Expectations, 19,* 1312–1323.

Chapter 5
Access to Primary Care and Preventive Health Services of LGBTQ+ Migrants, Refugees, and Asylum Seekers

Yudit Namer and Oliver Razum

5.1 Introduction

The Lancet issued calls to the international health community for taking urgent and solid steps towards "meeting the unique health-care needs of LGBTQ people" (2016a) as well as the right to health of refugee and migrant populations (2016b) in subsequent editorials, addressing primary care and preventative health services around the world. Refugees and asylum seekers represent the most vulnerable subgroup of the very heterogeneous migrant population. Non-heterosexual and/or non-cisgender identity contributes to this vulnerability, specifically in terms of access to healthcare. This chapter reviews the literature in advocacy of bridging the research and policy gap between the primary and preventive health services required by and the services provided for this specific group of migrants: LGBTQ+ refugees, and asylum seekers.

This chapter uses the abbreviation LGBTQ+ to refer to non-heterosexual and/or non-cisgender and questioning persons. The "+" in the abbreviation connotes an intentional inclusion. Terminology is clarified below for the unfamiliar. However, it should be noted that the political movements and the communities formed by non-heterosexual and/or non-cisgender individuals have historically assumed various abbreviations (e.g., GLB, LGBT, LGBTT, LGBTI, LGBTQIA) based on the inclusiveness of the political movements and the communities represented.

Y. Namer (✉) · O. Razum
Bielefeld University, School of Public Health, Department of Epidemiology & International Public Health, Bielefeld, Germany
e-mail: yudit.namer@uni-bielefeld.de

© The Author(s), under exclusive licence to Springer International Publishing AG, part of Springer Nature 2018
A. Rosano (ed.), *Access to Primary Care and Preventative Health Services of Migrants*, SpringerBriefs in Public Health, https://doi.org/10.1007/978-3-319-73630-3_5

LGBTQ+ Terminology

Transgender: Person whose gender identity and sex are not aligned. Can be used as 'trans' when referring to individuals. When transgender individuals' gender is needed to be referred to, their gender identity (the gender they experience) is used (e.g., trans man).

Cisgender: Person whose gender identity and sex are aligned. Can be used as 'cis' when referring to individuals (e.g., cis woman).

Lesbian: (Trans or cis) woman who is attracted to (trans or cis) women.

Gay: Person who is attracted to persons of their own gender. Also used to solely refer to (trans or cis) men who are attracted to (trans or cis) men.

Bisexual: Person who is attracted to persons of their own gender and another gender.

Intersex: Person whose sex differs from binary categories of sex due to variant developments of primary and secondary sex characteristics.

Queer: Person who does not identify within gender-binary and/or heteronormative categories.

Questioning: Person who is currently exploring their gender identity and/or sexual orientation.

+ This list by no means attempts to reduce gender identity and sexual orientation to categories, nor claims to be exhaustive. It is solely created for the purposes of following the arguments in the chapter, based on common usage by international LGBTQ+ civil society. An individual should always be asked how they define their gender and sexual orientation if referring to these attributes is necessary.

5.2   LGBTQ+ Population

Four percent of the US adults and 6% of EU respondents identify as LGBT[1] in surveys; probably an underestimate due to under-reporting (Dalia Research 2016; Gates 2017). Those born between 1980 and 1998, for example, are two times more likely to report identifying as LGBT than older generations in the US (Gates 2017). Respondents are also more likely to report identifying as LGBT when asked online, rather than in face-to-face interviews; and more likely to respond positively to having had any same-sex experience rather than identifying as LGB (Burkill et al. 2016). Difficulties in gathering data from non-US, non-EU countries suggest similar, if not greater problems in under-reporting due to political climates necessitating suppression, but do not imply that population proportions are different. Given the many ways in which people can experience their gender identity and/or sexual orientation, the developments within one's subjective expression of their identity,

---

[1] Identification as queer and/or intersex has not been largely surveyed.

and the societal climates within which these identities emerge, it is difficult to enumerate the LGBTQ+ population.

5.2.1 LGBTQ+ Refugee and Asylum Seekers

Asylum in the EU can be sought on the grounds of persecution due to sexual orientation and gender identity as legislated since 2004 and 2011, respectively. However, asylum on the grounds of gender expression (for individuals who do not conform to cultural perceptions of gender) and sex characteristics (for intersex individuals) are still not protected by legislation in the EU (International Lesbian, Gay, Bisexual, Trans and Intersex Association [ILGA] 2016a). Furthermore, due to the urgency of discretion, LGBTQ+ refugees and asylum seekers may choose to pursue protection on different grounds than gender identity and/or sexual orientation, such as political membership (ILGA 2016b).

Data regarding asylum claims on the grounds of sexual orientation or gender identity, thus how many LGBTQ+ refugees and asylum seekers currently reside in Europe are not reported (European Union Agency for Fundamental Rights 2017). The circumstances and the experiences of LGBTQ+ refugees and asylum seekers, however, are increasingly documented. As of May 2017, same-sex sexual activity is de facto illegal in 72 states around the world, in four of which the death penalty is applied as punishment. Death penalty for same-sex sexual relations is also reported in some non-sovereign, non-state regions. Similar sanctions exist for nonconforming gender expression (Carroll and Mendos 2017).

ILGA (2016b), summarizing the observations of human rights organizations and LGBTQ+ activists, details the following difficulties that LGBTQ+ refugees and asylum seekers experience: The rights to privacy and dignity are not always observed in asylum processes. Although questions regarding specific sexual practices are forbidden by the EU Court of Justice, these questions are still posed in certain asylum assessments. Authorities and administrative personnel involved in asylum procedures may lack information about gender identity and sexual orientation, countries of origin; or may lack sensitivity and awareness regarding the stigmatization in countries of origin (ILGA 2016b). Asylum procedures may even require the 'authentication' of asylum seekers' sexual orientation or gender identity by an LGBTQ+ organization in the region (Shakhsari 2014). Such practices may lead to unjust asylum rejections as applicants are not considered credibly LGBTQ+ based on stereotypes regarding gender and identity. Several states considered safe, either as a country of origin or as a third country to return refugees to, criminalize same-sex sexual activity or gender nonconformity. Considering the cases where LGBTQ+ asylum seekers have not yet disclosed sexual orientation and/or gender identity as their reason to flee, the return practices can be especially grave (ILGA 2016b). In addition, reception centres and camps in Turkey and EU member states are at times unsafe spaces where discrimination and violence in the shape of bullying, harassment and threat of physical and/or sexual abuse are observed (UNHCR 2015). Health services is one other area where a sense of safety is not ensured.

5.3 Specific Health Concerns

Data on the health of LGBTQ+ populations from Europe are scarce; findings regarding LGBTQ+ refugees and asylum seekers are scarcer (Keygnaert et al. 2014). Therefore, most findings outlined here will come from North American studies, and in cases, be adapted for LGBTQ+ refugees and asylum seekers.

5.3.1 HIV/AIDS

The first health issue that is most commonly associated with LGBTQ+ communities is HIV/AIDS. There are certain advantages and disadvantages to this bias. The obvious advantage is that LGBTQ+ communities receive a certain level of attention regarding HIV prevention. Many prevention programs are funded to target the communities, and many LGBTQ+ nongovernmental organizations have divisions focusing on HIV prevention. The downside is that LGBTQ+ communities are often pictured as high-risk, contributing to societies' stigmatization stance. In fact, Flowers (2001) argues that a collective 'otherization' of gay men, implying that 'at-risk'ness is an inherent part of being gay, has historically taken place in HIV/AIDS risk management and reductions efforts. In other words, societies used HIV/AIDS to create an artificial boundary between gay men and other members of their community, perceiving non-gay identities as superior, and gay identities as subordinate. On a different note of othering, Lombardi (2007) shows that trans men specifically feel invisible when it comes to HIV/AIDS prevention programs.

Nevertheless, disproportionately high rates of HIV transmission among men who have sex with men prevail. The European Centre for Disease Prevention and Control [ECDC] (2015) reports sexual activity between men to lead in HIV transmission rates in the EU and the European Economic Area, with the rates having increased again in the last 10 years. Similarly, UNAIDS (2016) reports a 17% increase in new diagnoses of HIV among men who have sex with men in western and central Europe. Furthermore, in 2014, 32% of new diagnoses were among migrants in Europe. Although transmission, according to a recent systematic review, often occurs post-migration, with migrant men who have sex with men more at risk (Fakoya et al. 2015), there is some evidence that suggests a mixture of colonial history, poverty, health inequity and social responses to HIV epidemics in the countries of origin plays a role in higher transmission rates among migrants (ECDC 2009).

5.3.2 Mental Health

Increased levels of suicidal ideation, depressive symptoms, anxiety, hypervigilance and posttraumatic symptoms have all been reported in LGBTQ+ individuals, in comparison with straight and cisgender counterparts (Alessi et al. 2013; Balsam et al. 2004; D'Augelli et al. 2002, 2006; Elliott et al. 2015; Matthews et al. 2002; Sandfort et al. 2006). For LGBTQ+ refugees and asylum seekers, mental health outlooks are even more intricate.

Alessi et al. (2016) recently explored the pre-migration experiences of LGBTQ+ asylees, refugees and persons with 'withholding of removal' status in Canada and the United States. What emerged from the interviews reflects the complexity of the LGBTQ+ refugees' and asylum seekers' circumstances: the participants reported fear of victimization by family members, community members, and the resultant hypervigilance to be a constant presence in their lives, even after being granted asylum. Practices to disguise gender identity and/or sexual orientation and to decrease visibility were constantly created and maintained to survive family- and community-level threats of victimization. Despite developing these strategies, victimization in the form of physical and sexual assault, crimes against significant others as well as property, threat and harassment, by members of the family, community, state authority or street gangs were reported to be routine. State actors specifically abused their role as protectors and were directly involved in acts of victimization (Alessi et al. 2016). Hate crimes against LGBTQ+ individuals are reported in all regions of the world, implying that LGBTQ+ refugees and asylum seekers, although possibly safer than in their country of origin, may not feel in an entirely safe environment in the host country. The UN High Commissioner for Human Rights (2011) reports gender-based lethal and non-lethal physical, sexual and psychological violence committed by religious and political extremists in the public sphere, and by family and community members in the private sphere, to be widespread global phenomena. Homophobic and transphobic acts of violence, some resulting in death, have been reported in all Council of Europe member states, providing ground for LGBTQ+ asylum seekers' prevailing hypervigilance in host countries (Council of Europe 2011).

Despite severe pre-migration and post-migration experiences of victimization, the resilience observed in LGBTQ+ refugees and asylum seekers is extensive. Alessi (2016) found that participants developed hope and maintained positivity as they grew increasingly free in their expression of gender identity and/or sexual orientation, even during times of isolation and ambiguity regarding status. Along with the support of friends and partners, community resources (most significantly mental health services, churches with LGBTQ+-inclusive services and legal aid) reinforced resilience, despite occasional conflicts. The participants also expressed that "doing whatever it takes" to survive in the host country as a refugee, including seeking transitional housing, social assistance, or employment below skill level demonstrated and reinforced their resilience. Finally, "giving back" to fellow LGBTQ+ refugees and asylum seekers in the forms of solidarity, advocacy and activism enhanced participants' resilience.

5.3.3 Gender-Conforming Processes

Not all transgender individuals prefer to go through medical gender-confirming procedures. For those individuals who do, hormone therapy may be the first, and in cases, sole step. The use of oestrogen or testosterone, depending on the person's gender identity should be facilitated by healthcare providers, as denying treatment usually leads to acquisition and unmonitored use of unregulated products with varying concentrations of sex hormones or anabolic steroids.

Endogenous puberty suppression procedures are becoming more frequent, with positive outcomes. Considering that gender identity is stable by the age of five, some medical professionals advocate for suppressing puberty to spare the child the distress of developing secondary sex characteristics which are incongruent with their gender identity (de Vries et al. 2011). It is likely that such options will be missed, not discussed by professionals, or not funded in the process of fleeing and seeking shelter in a new country with a healthcare system whose functioning is initially often not transparent to those in need.

5.4 Explaining Health Disparities Experienced by LGBTQ+ Populations

There are a number of models which have been utilized to explain health disparities that LGBTQ+ populations experience such as the Stress Process Model (Pearlin et al. 1981), or the Psychological Mediation Framework (Hatzenbuehler 2009). The current subchapter focuses on the Minority Stress Model as it is one of the first health models adapted to explore the LGBTQ+ experience, and the Health Equity Promotion Model, as it incorporates multilevel factors to explain the health outcomes of LGBTQ+ individuals.

5.4.1 The Minority Stress Model

According to this model, the continuous macro-level and micro-level stresses and victimizations minorities face daily, connoting a culturally perceived inferiority, negatively impact individuals' immune system and deem them more vulnerable to certain ailments, compared to the members of the majority population (Brooks 1981). As a 'sexual minority', LGB individuals, in response to systemic barriers, may go through objective as well as subjective processes of acute and continuous discrimination, resultant hypervigilance based on anticipation of discrimination, internalization of discriminatory attitudes towards self, and disguise of identity (Meyer 2013). Although this model was initially articulated in reference to LGB individuals, it is argued to aptly denote the experiences of transgender and gender nonconforming persons as well (Hendricks and Testa 2012). The negative effect may be increased if a second discriminating factor such as asylum seeker status is present.

5.4.2   The Health Equity Promotion Model

Fredriksen-Goldsen et al. (2014) argue for a more comprehensive exploration of LGBTQ+ health which takes a life course approach, considering risks but also resiliences of the LGBTQ+ populations. This model focuses on the human right to health and where responsibilities lie to ensure it. Specifically, the model reflects on how LGBTQ+ individuals' health outcomes are impacted by the intersections between their social positions in terms of age, ethnicity and socioeconomic status; the context they are in, individually, environmentally and structurally; and the bio-psycho-social processes by which health is promoted.

If we were to consider LGBTQ+ refugees and asylum seekers from the super-diversity perspective, this model appears to more fully encompass the unique intersectionality of being a sexual as well as ethnic and/or religious minority. Vertovec (2007), in a seminal anthropological contribution, argued that the global migration patterns in the last decades have generated societal conditions of super-diversity, an increasing diversification of legal status, ethnicity, languages spoken and being learnt, skills brought and religions practised, among others. Super-diversity shapes societal discourses by being both invited and resisted against. It can even be said that openness to super-diversity defines the nature of a society. Gender identity, gender expression, sexual orientation and their conformance to dominant societal norms are increasingly becoming part of the diversity narrative of today's migration patterns due to the visibility efforts of activists and resultant gradual disappearance of identity suppressing mechanisms in parts of the world.

An LGBTQ+ individual, who was prosecuted for their gender identity and/or sexual orientation in their home country may experience a decrease in perceived discrimination due to gender identity and/or sexual orientation, yet find themselves increasingly discriminated against due to their social positions determined by residency status, nationality, religion or language. The person has to continually adapt and respond to the challenges and opportunities put forward by the host society. One specific challenge is access to primary care and preventive health services.

5.5   Access to Primary Care and Preventive Health Services

5.5.1   Migrants', Refugees' and Asylum Seekers' Access to Primary Care and Preventive Health Services

Migrants with various residency statuses face certain barriers in accessing primary and preventive health services. Variance in entitlements across Europe complicates the picture. In Germany, for example, access to healthcare is initially restricted for arriving asylum seekers and refugees in both legal and administrative terms. Specifically, asylum seekers waiting for status; who hold a temporary residence permit on humanitarian grounds; whose application for political asylum is denied but repatriation is awaiting; and who are awaiting expulsion due to rejection of asylum application are only entitled to access treatment for emergencies, acute and painful ailments, pregnancy care, vaccinations and preventative measures when necessary. Other treatment might be granted by the local welfare agency only on a case-by-case basis. Individuals can access the restricted services via healthcare vouchers in most of the federal states, obtaining of which can be a repetitive and confusing process. The waiting time for full entitlement to healthcare to be granted is 15 months (Bozorgmehr and Razum 2015).

Culturally inappropriate interventions, lack of diversity training in service providing staff, language barriers in terms of lack of service providers offering services in the client's language as well as administrative difficulties in recruiting an interpreter further impede access to care (Razum and Bozorgmehr 2016). Lack of trust in the host country's system structures add to access barriers (Majumder et al. 2015). Refugees and asylum seekers, whose cases are pending, often report their choice of not seeing UNHCR-referred health practitioners out of fear that their health details will be shared with the UNHCR officials and the third country of asylum (Shakhsari 2014).

5.5.2   LGBTQ+ Refugees' and Asylum Seekers' Access to Primary Care and Preventive Health Services

As the categories become narrower, the uniqueness of challenges, and needs for solutions proportionally increase. A key study by the UNHCR (2015) revealed that 63% of their offices which engage in organizing or funding healthcare were aware of working with LGBTQ+ individuals. Out of government partners of the UNHCR, 5% provided hormone therapy for transgender service users, 7% provided mental health and LGBTQ + −related psychosocial support, and 21% provided treatment for HIV/AIDS. The study emphasizes the significance of nongovernmental partners since 7% provided hormone therapy, 28% HIV/AIDS treatment, 30% mental health support and 40% LGBTQ + −related psychosocial support.

One of the most comprehensive qualitative studies on this issue surveyed LGBTQ+ refugees and asylum seekers from Iran, based in Turkey, waiting to hear about their asylum application status. Although all refugees and asylum seekers have access to primary healthcare in Turkey, the study showed that LGBTQ+ refugees and asylum seekers faced unique barriers. Specifically, the study participants indicated that they were subjected to intrusive personal questions by healthcare workers irrelevant to their health upon revealing their sexual orientation and/or gender identity. Transgender individuals who wished to initiate or resume gender-confirming medical processes, that is, procedures to align their bodies with their gender identity, such as affirmative hormone treatment, reported that the primary healthcare physicians were often unknowledgeable about gender-confirmation and that hormones, when prescribed, were often financially out of reach (Kara and Çalık 2016).

Language and cultural barriers are experienced on different layers by LGBTQ+ refugees and asylum seekers: healthcare providers may lack the appropriate sexual orientation/gender identity vocabulary in addition to their unfamiliarity with the individuals' cultural background and language of origin. Making interpretation services available does not by itself ameliorate the issue; interpreters are not always acquainted with standards of care in providing services to LGBTQ+ individuals (Emanvel 2016). This barrier, as it muddles personal narrative, is specifically distressing in mental healthcare. Kara and Çalık's (2016) participants reported that the mental healthcare they received was complicated by the use of interpreters, and mental health professionals' lack of expertise in LGBTQ+ issues. They further described the available care as medicalized, that is, more inclined to comprise of psychopharmacology than psychotherapy. Due to the low number of professionals available, the consultations were months apart from each other.

When challenges of accessing healthcare as an LGBTQ+ individual such as the lack of LGBTQ + −ally practices or othering prevention management stances are coupled with the restricted entitlements and structural access barriers for refugees and asylum seekers, acute and chronic health problems will be left untreated, and the individual will be open to certain health risks. The restoration and promotion of health equity in the case of LGBTQ+ refugees and asylum seekers fall on policymakers, service providers, as well as the community at large.

5.6   Recommendations

A recent study by Kahn et al. (2017) exploring the perceptions of service providers working with LGBTQ+ refugees and asylum seekers in Canada concluded that the services should first ensure that a sense of safety is built. Although a sense of safety is essential for all interactions between service users and providers, the participants in this study underscored the centrality of safety and trust for the care LGBTQ+ refugees and asylum seekers, who are survivors of lifelong of victimization. Furthermore, recognition of the idiosyncrasies of needs and challenges was identified as a promoter of wellbeing. Negotiating personal biases regarding identities was also expressed as essential to provide the best possible care to LGBTQ+ refugees and asylum seekers.

In the light of the findings summarized in this chapter, we propose not LGBTQ + −specific services, nor any form of segregation for migrant populations, but for regular services to become increasingly migrant− and LGBTQ + −sensitive. A diversity management approach would ensure the diversification of service providers, services provided, and user needs to achieve this goal. This chapter builds on this premise and offers the following recommendation to policy makers and service providers.

5.6.1 Recommendations to Policymakers for LGBTQ+ Ally Service Provision

Lift all access barriers to primary and preventive healthcare Access to healthcare is a human right, and neither residency status, nor gender identity and sexual orientation should be used as a pretext to limit rights. Yet, in addition to restricted entitlements in parts of Europe, language and cultural barriers reduce refugees' and asylum seekers' access to healthcare (Razum and Bozorgmehr 2016) with LGBTQ+ identity acting as an additional barrier between the right to healthcare and the care provided. As Feldman (2006) summarizes, complete access to preventive and primary mental and physical healthcare as well as access to translation and interpretation services, specialist services for survivors of violence and information about these services in relevant languages should be granted to all refugees and asylum seekers.

Educate about gender identity, sexual orientation and their expressions It is important to face one's biases regarding how gender and orientation are expressed. Not all users of gynaecological health services identify as woman, and transgender women can have prostate cancer, for example. Most importantly, it is of importance not to assume someone's gender identity and/or sexual orientation by their expression. Not assuming the gender of someone's romantic or sexual partner, and in terms of non-cisgender identity, asking the person's preferred pronoun to refer to them are components of best practice. Such knowledge, by policy, should be part of the training of all parties involved in health systems, from care providers to researchers.

5.6.2 Recommendations to Service Providers for Advocacy-Based Service Provision

'Come out' to service users Not only should primary healthcare workers be educated about LGBTQ+ issues, as well as difficulties faced by refugees and asylum seekers, but the insight garnered should be visible. One tool for visibility is to place a rainbow flag, a prominent symbol of LGBTQ+ community, to reduce the fear of using the services, and to communicate alliance.

Design an LGBTQ+ ally practice Build a team comprised of healthcare workers and interpreters of several languages. One aspect of an LGBTQ+ ally practice, for example, is de-genderizing bathrooms. Anecdotal experiences with patients suggest that transgender individuals avoid health services altogether out of the fear that they will be asked for a urine sample, without offering the use of a suitable, gender-neutral bathroom. Ask the users how to better design safer spaces.

Recognize family connections which may not be legally recognized The intersectionality of being LGBTQ+ as well as refugee or asylum seeker leads to various family constellations. It is important to recognize that LGBTQ+ refugees and asylum seekers may have spouses that are not recognized by national laws of the host country or the country of origin, or may not be biologically related to their children whom they co-parent with their partners and/or family members.

Recognize the LGBTQ+ migrant, refugee and asylum seeker social networks in your region These networks are not only the referral points for LGBTQ+ migrants, refugees and asylum seekers who may be feeling isolated in a new land, removed from their existing social networks; they are also great resources to receive training for LGBTQ+ issues.

References

Alessi, E. J. (2016). Resilience in sexual and gender minority forced migrants: A qualitative exploration. *Traumatology, 22*, 203–213. https://doi.org/10.1037/trm0000077

Alessi, E. J., Martin, J. I., Gyamerah, A., & Meyer, I. H. (2013). Prejudice events and traumatic stress among heterosexuals and lesbians, gay men and bisexuals. *Journal of Aggression, Maltreatment & Trauma, 22*, 510–526. https://doi.org/10.1080/10926771.2013.785455

Alessi, E. J., Kahn, S., & van der Horn, R. (2016). A qualitative exploration of the premigration victimization experiences of sexual and gender minority refugees and asylees in the United States and Canada. *The Journal of Sex Research, 54*, 1–13. https://doi.org/10.1080/00224499.2016.1229738

Balsam, K. F., Huang, B., Fieland, K. C., Simoni, J. M., & Walters, K. L. (2004). Culture, trauma, and wellness: A comparison of heterosexual and lesbian, gay, bisexual, and two-spirit Native Americans. *Cultural Diversity and Ethnic Minority Psychology, 10*, 287–301. https://doi.org/10.1037/1099-9809.10.3.287

Brooks, V. R. (1981). Minority stress and lesbian women. Lexington, MA: Lexington Books.

Bozorgmehr, K., & Razum, O. (2015). Effect of restricting access to health care on health expenditures among asylum-seekers and refugees: A quasi-experimental study in Germany, 1994–2013. *PLoS One, 10*, e0131483. https://doi.org/10.1371/journal.pone.0131483

Burkill, S., Copas, A., Couper, M. P., Clifton, S., Prah, P., Datta, J., et al. (2016). Using the web to collect data on sensitive behaviours: A study looking at mode effects on the British national survey of sexual attitudes and lifestyles. *PLoS One, 11*, e0147983. https://doi.org/10.1371/journal.pone.0147983

Carroll, A., & Mendos, L. R. (2017). State sponsored homophobia 2017. http://ilga.org/downloads/2017/ILGA_State_Sponsored_Homophobia_2017_WEB.pdf. Accessed 24 Jul 2017.

Council of Europe. (2011). *Discrimination on grounds of sexual orientation and gender identity in Europe* (2nd ed.). Strasbourg: Council of Europe Publishing.

D'Augelli, A. R., Pilkington, N. W., & Hershberger, S. L. (2002). Incidence and mental health impact of sexual orientation victimization of lesbian, gay, and bisexual youths in high school. *School Psychology Quarterly, 17*, 148–167. https://doi.org/10.1521/scpq.17.2.148.20854

D'Augelli, A. R., Grossman, A. H., & Starks, M. T. (2006). Childhood gender atypicality, victimization, and PTSD among lesbian, gay, and bisexual youth. *Journal of Interpersonal Violence, 21*, 1462–1482. https://doi.org/10.1177/0886260506293482

Dalia Research. (2016). Counting the LGBT population: 6% of Europeans identify as LGBT. https://daliaresearch.com/counting-the-lgbt-population-6-of-europeans-identify-as-lgbt/. Accessed 13 Sept 2017.

de Vries A. L. C., Steensma, T. D., Doreleijers, T. A. H., & Cohen-Kettenis, P. T. (2011). Puberty suppression in adolescents with gender identity disorder: A prospective follow-up study. *The Journal of Sexual Medicine, 8*, 2276–2283. https://doi.org/10.1111/j.1743-6109.2010.01943.x

Elliott, M. N., Kanouse, D. E., Burkhart, Q., Abel, G. A., Lyratzopoulos, G., Beckett, M. K., et al. (2015). Sexual minorities in England have poorer health and worse health care experiences: A national survey. *Journal of General Internal Medicine, 30*, 9–16. https://doi.org/10.1007/s11606-014-2905-y

Emanvel, B. (2016). The difficulties of being an LGBT refugee in Germany. http://wafmag.org/2016/06/difficulties-lgbt- refugee-germany/. Accessed 10 Oct 2016.

European Centre for Disease Prevention and Control. (2009). *Migrant health: Epidemiology of HIV and AIDS in migrant communities and ethnic minorities in EU/EEA countries*. Stockholm: ECDC.

European Centre for Disease Prevention and Control, & WHO Regional Office for Europe. (2015). *HIV/AIDS surveillance in Europe 2014*. Stockholm: ECDC.

European Union Agency for Fundamental Rights. (2017). Current migration situation in the EU: Lesbian, gay, bisexual, transgender and intersex asylum seekers. http://fra.europa.eu/sites/default/files/fra_uploads/fra-march-2017-monthly-migration-report-focus-lgbti_en.pdf. Accessed 21 July 2017.

Fakoya, I., Álvarez-del Arco, D., Woode-Owusu, M., Monge, S., Rivero-Montesdeoca, Y., Delpech, V., et al. (2015). A systematic review of post-migration acquisition of HIV among migrants from countries with generalised HIV epidemics living in Europe: Implications for effectively managing HIV prevention programmes and policy. *BMC Public Health, 15*, 561. https://doi.org/10.1186/s12889-015-1852-9

Feldman, R. (2006). Primary health care for refugees and asylum seekers: A review of the literature and a framework for services. *Public Health, 120*, 809–816. https://doi.org/10.1016/j.puhe.2006.05.014

Flowers, P. (2001). Gay men and HIV/AIDS risk management. *Health, 5*, 50–75.

Fredriksen-Goldsen, K. I., Simoni, J. M., Kim, H.-J., Lehavot, K., Walters, K. L., Yang, J., et al. (2014). The health equity promotion model: Reconceptualization of lesbian, gay, bisexual, and transgender (LGBT) health disparities. *American Journal of Orthopsychiatry, 84*, 653–663. https://doi.org/10.1037/ort0000030

Gates, G. J. (2017). In US, more adults identifying as LGBT. http://www.gallup.com/poll/201731/lgbt-identification-rises.aspx. Accessed 21 July 2017.

Hatzenbuehler, M. L. (2009). How does sexual minority stigma "get under the skin"? A psychological mediation framework. *Psychological Bulletin, 135*, 707–730. https://doi.org/10.1037/a0016441

Hendricks, M. L., & Testa, R. J. (2012). A conceptual framework for clinical work with transgender and gender nonconforming clients: An adaptation of the Minority Stress Model. *Professional Psychology: Research and Practice, 43*, 460–467. https://doi.org/10.1037/a0029597

International Lesbian, Gay, Bisexual, Trans and Intersex Association [ILGA]. (2016a). Protecting the rights of LGBTI asylum seekers and refugees in the reform of the common European asylum system. https://www.ilga-europe.org/sites/default/files/Attachments/ilga-europe_-_protecting_the_rights_of_lgbti_asylum_seekers_and_refugees_in_the_ceas_-_december_2016.pdf. Accessed 21 July 2017.

International Lesbian, Gay, Bisexual, Trans and Intersex Association [ILGA]. (2016b). Seeking refuge without harassment, detention or return to a "safe country". https://www.ilga-europe.org/sites/default/files/Attachments/ilga_europe_briefing_on_lgbti_asylum_issues_-_february_2016.pdf. Accessed 21 July 2017.

Kahn, S., Alessi, E., Woolner, L., Kim, H., & Olivieri, C. (2017). Promoting the wellbeing of lesbian, gay, bisexual and transgender forced migrants in Canada: Providers' perspectives. *Culture, Health & Sexuality, 19*, 1165–1179. https://doi.org/10.1080/13691058.2017.1298843

Kara, H., & Çalık, D. (2016). *"Tekin olmayi" beklerken: LGBTİ mültecilerin ara durağı Türkiye.* Ankara: KAOS GL.

Keygnaert, I., Guieu, A., Ooms, G., Vettenburg, N., Temmerman, M., & Roelens, K. (2014). Sexual and reproductive health of migrants: Does the EU care? *Health Policy, 114*, 215–225. https://doi.org/10.1016/j.healthpol.2013.10.007

Lombardi, E. (2007). Public health and trans-people: Barriers to care and strategies to improve treatment. In I. H. Meyer & M. E. Northridge (Eds.), *The health of sexual minorities* (pp. 638–652). Boston: Springer US. https://doi.org/10.1007/978-0-387-31334-4_26

Majumder, P., O'Reilly, M., Karim, K., & Vostanis, P. (2015). 'This doctor, I not trust him, I'm not safe': the perceptions of mental health and services by unaccompanied refugee adolescents. *The International Journal of Social Psychiatry, 61*, 129–136. https://doi.org/10.1177/0020764014537236

Matthews, A. K., Hughes, T. L., Johnson, T., Razzano, L. A., & Cassidy, R. (2002). Prediction of depressive distress in a community sample of women: The role of sexual orientation. *American Journal of Public Health, 92*, 1131–1139. https://doi.org/10.2105/AJPH.92.7.1131

Meyer, I. H. (2013). Prejudice, social stress, and mental health in lesbian, gay, and bisexual populations: conceptual issues and research evidence. *Psychology of Sexual Orientation and Gender Diversity, 1*(S), 3–26. https://doi.org/10.1037/2329-0382.1.S.3

Pearlin, L. I., Menaghan, E. G., Lieberman, M. A., & Mullan, J. T. (1981). The stress process. *Journal of Health and Social Behavior, 22*, 337–356. https://doi.org/10.2307/2136676

Razum, O., & Bozorgmehr, K. (2016). Restricted entitlements and access to health care for refugees and immigrants: The example of Germany. *Global Social Policy, 16*, 321–324. https://doi.org/10.1177/1468018116655267

Sandfort, T. G. M., Bakker, F., Schellevis, F. G., & Vanwesenbeeck, I. (2006). Sexual orientation and mental and physical health status: Findings from a Dutch population survey. *American Journal of Public Health, 96*, 1119–1125. https://doi.org/10.2105/AJPH.2004.058891

Shakhsari, S. (2014). The queer time of death: Temporality, geopolitics, and refugee rights. *Sexualities, 17*, 998–1015. https://doi.org/10.1177/1363460714552261

The Lancet. (2016a). Meeting the unique health-care needs of LGBTQ people. *The Lancet, 387*, 95. https://doi.org/10.1016/S0140-6736(16)00013-1

The Lancet. (2016b). Refugee and migrant crisis: The deficient global response. *The Lancet, 388*, 633. https://doi.org/10.1016/S0140-6736(16)31342-3

UN High Commissioner for Human Rights. (2011). Discriminatory laws and practices and acts of violence against individuals based on their sexual orientation and gender identity. http://www.ohchr.org/Documents/Issues/Discrimination/A.HRC.19.41_English.pdf. Accessed 13 Sept 2017.

UN High Commissioner for Refugees (UNHCR). (2015). Protecting persons with diverse sexual orientations and gender identities: A global report on UNHCR's efforts to protect lesbian, gay, bisexual, transgender, and intersex Asylum-Seekers and refugees. http://reliefweb.int/sites/reliefweb.int/files/resources/566140454.pdf. Accessed 24 July 2017.

UNAIDS. (2016). *Prevention gap report.* Geneva: UNAIDS.

Vertovec, S. (2007). Super-diversity and its implications. *Ethnic and Racial Studies, 30*, 1024–1054. https://doi.org/10.1080/01419870701599465

Chapter 6
Health-Related Lifestyles Among Migrants in Europe

Teresa Spadea, Raffaella Rusciani, Luisa Mondo, and Giuseppe Costa

6.1 Introduction

Differences in health related lifestyles can explain part of the difference in health outcomes between immigrant and host populations, as well as across different migrant groups. Characterizing the risk profile of migrant populations is therefore essential in order to prioritize actions for prevention and health services organization. The mechanisms that affect the occurrence of risky behaviours among immigrants are very complex, depending on the interrelation between two broad groups of health determinants: individual and contextual cultural and socioeconomic factors, on one side; and migration characteristics, particularly country of origin, age at arrival and length of residence, on the other side. The scientific literature on health related lifestyles and risk factors for chronic diseases among immigrants, however, does not systematically account for these complex mechanisms.

This chapter will try to systematize the available knowledge, starting with a brief conceptual framework of the mechanisms underlying the relationship between migration and health, and then focusing on a synthetic review of the existing literature on the main health related lifestyles (i.e. diet, physical activity, smoking and cardiovascular risk factors) and their determinants.

T. Spadea (✉) · R. Rusciani · L. Mondo
Epidemiology Unit, ASL TO3 Piedmont Region, Grugliasco, TO, Italy
e-mail: teresa.spadea@epi.piemonte.it

G. Costa
Department of Clinical and Biological Sciences, University of Turin, Turin,
Italy and Epidemiology Unit, ASL TO3 Piedmont Region, Grugliasco, TO, Italy

© The Author(s), under exclusive licence to Springer International Publishing AG,
part of Springer Nature 2018
A. Rosano (ed.), *Access to Primary Care and Preventative Health Services of Migrants*,
SpringerBriefs in Public Health, https://doi.org/10.1007/978-3-319-73630-3_6

6.2   The Conceptual Framework

The health profile of migrants can be determined by three main categories of determinants and related health problems: importation diseases, uprooting effects and health consequences of acculturation and social inequalities. The relative importance of each of these three classes of health problems varies with time since migration.

6.2.1   Importation Diseases

This group includes health conditions with a genetic basis and infectious diseases endemic in the country of origin, e.g. tuberculosis or HIV, which are usually detected soon after the migrant arrival. In some cases, however, infectious agents may have long-term consequences: it is the case of some cancers of viral origin, such as stomach cancer associated with *Helicobacter Pylori*, liver cancer with chronic hepatitis or cervical cancer with the *Human Papilloma Virus*. These are in fact the more common cancers in less developed countries, with higher incidence than in western societies (Ferlay 2013), which have been also found among immigrants in Europe (Arnold 2010).

Although the import of infectious diseases is often considered an alarming public health problem for the host population, these diseases do not represent a significant share of the burden of illness of foreign immigrants.

6.2.2   Uprooting Effects

In the short-term, the migration experience and the resulting uprooting phenomenon can have a direct negative impact on psychological wellbeing and mental health, including the initiation of risky behaviours such as smoking, alcohol or substance abuse. A high prevalence of depression has been observed particularly among young immigrants who had experienced traumas in their originating countries (Pfarrwaller e Suris 2012), as in the case of refugees and asylum seekers. High levels of mental health problems have been reported in detained asylum seekers, with persistent negative effects even after the release (Robjant 2009). Refugees and asylum seekers, however, although increasing in recent years, still represent a very small percentage of the immigrant population living in Europe.

6.2.3 Acculturation and Social Inequalities

Acculturation and social inequalities have the major impact on the long term. Acculturation, which is in general a process where two cultures interact and integrate within each other, shows its impact on health through the progressive adaptation of migrants to the habits of the host country. Several studies have consistently shown that health related behaviours and their consequent health outcomes vary according to the country of origin, with its culture and traditions; age at arrival, with a faster process among younger migrants and workers, who are more likely to be in contact with the native population at school or in workplaces; and length of residence in the host country (McKay et al. 2003). This phenomenon, in turn, is mediated by the individual socioeconomic position of migrants, as well as by contextual factors in both origin and host countries (Nazroo 2003; Malmusi et al. 2010; Acevedo-Garcia 2012). In the large majority of the cases, in fact, migrants have a low socioeconomic status at arrival and tend to cumulate social disadvantages with time. This implies that also their behaviours tend to assimilate to those of the lowest socioeconomic groups of the host population, usually resulting in an increase in risky behaviours (Lara et al. 2005). At the same time, migrants usually benefit from better health care and hygiene conditions in the host country and therefore experience a decrease in morbidity from infectious diseases and in maternal and infant mortality, while shifting towards the epidemiological profile of western countries, with an increase in risks of chronic diseases.

Finally, the epidemiological profile of migrants is also altered by two typical selection mechanisms that may bias the association between migration and health, namely the "healthy migrant effect" and the "salmon (or remigration) bias" (Razum et al. 2000; Razum 2006; Ulmann et al. 2011). The first effect assumes that only individuals who are particularly healthy choose to leave their countries and seek better life conditions abroad; the second hypothesis suggests that older or ill migrants tend to remigrate to their countries of origin to live the last part of their life in a more familiar environment. Both imply an underestimation of the morbidity and mortality of migrants, since sicker individuals would stay or return to their countries and data on their health outcomes are usually not available.

This framework shows clearly that migrants' health is determined by a variety of exposures and contextual factors, operating in different phases of their life, and only a life course approach that takes into account the whole migration process could provide new knowledge on the health profile of migrants (Spallek 2011). Moreover, it is worth noting that the health problems of migrants are not exclusively associated with migration itself: importation diseases may be the same for travellers, as well as uprooting effects are similar in all tragic life events (such as bereavement or loss of work) and social inequalities in health are shared with the whole population. However, in the case of migration, these mechanisms interact with other experiences that potentially generate new and stronger inequalities, such as racial discrimination, cultural difficulties or legal constraints (Nazroo 2003, Scheppers et al.

2006; Hacker et al. 2015): all these factors represent important barriers to the preservation of the migrants' health capital, which should be effectively countered.

6.3   Data from the Literature

We searched MEDLINE for articles on health behaviours and life styles among immigrants in Europe, published in English from 2000 to June 2017. We ended with 48 papers, judged more pertinent to our objectives. However, due to space constraints, we will not report here the complete list of references, but we will try to synthesize the most interesting and consistent results.

The vast majority of articles focussed on diet, physical activity and overweight. The results highlight great ethnic variability in all these behaviours, depending mostly on the origin culture and socioeconomic factors, as well as on the characteristics of the migratory process. For example, as far as culture of origin is concerned, the observance of the Muslim religious prohibition of drinking alcoholics may have an important role in the very low alcohol consumption rates generally observed among migrants (Mejean et al. 2007; Hansen et al. 2008; Carrasco-Garrido et al. 2009; Bodenmann et al. 2010). One study found that a strong barrier to changes towards a healthier diet among Pakistani women in Norway was represented by the social dimension of food, with strong expectations from men and children for rich and fat meals during social gatherings (Raberg Kjollesdal et al. 2010). Qualitative studies emphasize the fatalistic approach to health of some ethnic minorities, particularly Gypsies or people from sub-Saharan Africa (Van Cleemput et al. 2007; Cooper et al. 2012): this implies low awareness of chronic diseases and a poor attitude towards health prevention. More generally, immigrants who tend to form close social networks, with a poor mix with natives, experience poorer health than those who live in open networks (Rostila 2010).

As said before, acculturation is a complex process that can have positive or negative effects on health, depending on both individual and contextual characteristics. While most of the papers show that longer durations of residence are accompanied by a deterioration of health, and in particular by an increase in weight mediated by the acquisition of unhealthy diet (Maqoud et al. 2016; Casali et al. 2015; Akbulut 2014; Garduno-Diaz and Khokhar 2013), Spanish studies find that a longer length of residence protect from overweight compared to both natives and recent immigrants (Esteban-Gonzalo et al. 2015; Marin-Guerrero et al. 2015). One possible explanation for this unexpected result is that immigrants in Spain are mostly from Latin America, an area with an increasing prevalence of obesity, and benefit from the transition to a healthier Mediterranean diet.

An important role in determining lifestyles is also played by socioeconomic factors, with higher educational levels and socioeconomic positions associated with healthier behaviours. Increased language proficiency, which in turn is associated with length of residence and acculturation, has been reported as a significant determinant of leisure time physical activity (Jonsson et al. 2013). Compared to other risk factors, physical activity in particular appears to be linked to cultural and economic factors (Gonzalez Lopez et al. 2015; Besharat Pour et al. 2014; Hansen et al. 2008), possibly because it might be perceived as a luxury rather than a need for health, particularly among females. In a recent Italian study (Loi 2017) inactive migrants appear to be protected from alcohol and smoking habits. This result is in line with the hypothesis that people outside the labour market would be less in contact with the host population and subject to a slower acculturation process, being therefore protected from taking unhealthy lifestyles. At the same time, however, it emerges a significant impact of two integration indicators, particularly among women: the sense of loneliness, which increases the risk of smoking, and language difficulties with the doctor, which are associated with greater obesity.

Another line of research focuses on the major risk factors for cardiovascular diseases (CVD), which, in addition to obesity discussed above, include smoking, hypertension, and diabetes. The relative difference in the CVD burden seems to depend mainly on ethnic origins and country of residence. However, as clearly pointed out by Agyemang et al. (2012), given the increasing prevalence of CVD in low income countries, it is difficult to disentangle the relative effect of imported risk factors from those acquired with time through the acculturation process, on one side; and from the role of contextual factors in the host country, including the health care system, the socioeconomic situation, or environmental factors, on the other side. More insight comes from the comparison of different ethnic groups in different contexts. Studies comparing ethnic minorities with the population remained in the country of origin generally show higher prevalence of CVD risk factors among migrants than among the same ethnic groups in their countries (Singh and Kirchengast 2011; Akbulut et al. 2014; Maqoud et al. 2016). The opposite was observed among Tunisian migrants in France, who showed lower levels of overweight, diabetes, smoking, hypertension and hypercholesterolemia as compared to both French and Tunisians living in Tunisia (Mejean et al. 2007). A possible explanation might be the combined effect of the continuation of healthy behavioural traditions (low alcohol consumption) along with better access to health services and a more active lifestyle. When comparing the same ethnic group after migration to different industrialized countries, results have a substantial variability by country of residence: for example, in a comparative analysis of CVD risk between English and Dutch immigrants, smoking was more frequent among migrants in the Netherlands than among the same ethnic groups in England, suggesting a relevant role of contextual factors (Agyemang et al. 2012).

6.4 Conclusions

The profile of the main unhealthy behaviours shows a less favourable situation for migrants than what is generally seen for mortality or morbidity thanks to the "healthy migrant effect". These data are alarming to those that could be their health outcomes in a few years: overweight and obesity might be predictors of metabolic syndrome and cardiovascular disease; lack of physical activity, apart from being a predictor of overweight, seems to be linked to poor mental health, with symptoms like anxiety and depression (Siddiqui et al. 2014).

Unhealthy lifestyles vary widely by ethnic group as a function of their culture of origin. Generally speaking, behaviours tend to worsen with the duration of stay, particularly among migrants in the lower socioeconomic groups, and are exacerbated by the sense of loneliness and low levels of integration in the host country.

A challenge for future research is to identify culturally sensitive interventions to facilitate healthy behaviours, so as to reinforce the positive effects of the acculturation process, while counteracting the possible adverse effects. More inclusion and integration policies are also needed to partially interrupt the deterioration of health capital that appears already in place in most countries and to prevent future mortality (Ikram 2015). At the same time, such policies should be accompanied by specific actions to support the most vulnerable socioeconomic groups.

References

Acevedo-Garcia, D., Sanchez-Vaznaugh, E. V., Viruell-Fuentes, E. A., & Almeida, J. (2012). Integrating social epidemiology into immigrant health research: A cross-national framework. *Social Science & Medicine, 75*, 2060–2068.

Agyemang, C., de-Graft Aikins, A., & Bhopal, R. (2012). Ethnicity and cardiovascular health research: Pushing the boundaries by including comparison populations in the countries of origin. *Ethnicity & Health, 17*, 579–596.

Akbulut, G., Yildirim, M., Sanlier, N., van Stralen, M. M., Acar-Tek, N., Bilici, S., et al. (2014). Comparison of energy balance-related behaviours and measures of body composition between Turkish adolescents in Turkey and Turkish immigrant adolescents in the Netherlands. *Public Health Nutrition, 17*, 2692–2699.

Arnold, M., Razum, O., & Coebergh, J. L. (2010). Cancer risk diversity in non-western migrants to Europe: An overview of the literature. *European Journal of Cancer, 46*, 2647–2659.

Besharat Pour, M., Bergstrom, A., Bottai, M., Kull, I., Wickman, M., Hakansson, N., et al. (2014). Effect of parental migration background on childhood nutrition, physical activity, and body mass index. *Journal of Obesity, 2014*, 406529.

Bodenmann, P., Cornuz, J., Vaucher, P., Ghali, W., Daeppen, J. B., & Favrat, B. (2010). A health behaviour cross-sectional study of immigrants and non-immigrants in a Swiss urban general-practice setting. *Journal of Immigrant and Minority Health, 12*, 24–32.

Carrasco-Garrido, P., Jimenez-Garcia, R., Barrera, V. H., de Andres, A. L., & de Miguel, A. G. (2009). Significant differences in the use of healthcare resources of native-born and foreign born in Spain. *BMC Public Health, 9*, 201.

Casali, M. E., Borsari, L., Marchesi, I., Borella, P., & Bargellini, A. (2015). Lifestyle and food habits changes after migration: A focus on immigrant women in Modena (Italy). *Annali di Igiene, 27*, 748–759.

Cooper, M., Harding, S., Mullen, K., & O'Donnell, C. (2012). 'A chronic disease is a disease which keeps coming back...It is like the flu': Chronic disease risk perception and explanatory models among French- and Swahili-speaking African migrants. *Ethnicity & Health, 17*, 597–613.

Esteban-Gonzalo, L., Veiga, O. L., Regidor, E., Martinez, D., Marcos, A., & Calle, M. E. (2015). Immigrant status. Acculturation and risk of overweight and obesity in adolescents living in Madrid (Spain): The AFINOS study. *Journal of Immigrant and Minority Health, 17*, 367–374.

Ferlay, J., Soerjomataram, I., Ervik, M., Dikshit, R., Eser, S., Mathers, C., et al. (2013). GLOBOCAN 2012 v1.0, Cancer Incidence and Mortality Worldwide: IARC CancerBase No. 11 [Internet]. Lyon, France: International Agency for Research on Cancer. Available from:http://globocan. iarc.fr/Pages/fact_sheets_cancer.aspx, accessed on 22/01/2018.

Garduno-Diaz, S. D., & Khokhar, S. (2013). South Asian dietary patterns and their association with risk factors for the metabolic syndrome. *Journal of Human Nutrition and Dietetics, 26*, 145–155.

Gonzalez-Lopez, J. R., Rodriguez-Gazquez Mde, L., & Lomas-Campos Mde, L. (2015). Physical activity in Latin American immigrant adults living in Seville, Spain. *Nursing Research, 64*, 476–484.

Hacker, K., Anies, M., Folb, B. L., & Zallman, L. (2015). Barriers to health care for undocumented immigrants: A literature review. *Risk Management and Healthcare Policy, 8*, 175–183.

Hansen, A. R., Ekholm, O., & Kjoller, M. (2008). Health behaviour among non-Western immigrants with Danish citizenship. *Scandinavian Journal of Public Health, 36*, 205–210.

Ikram, U. Z., Malmusi, D., Juel, K., Rey, G., & Kunst, A. E. (2015). Association between integration policies and immigrants' mortality: An explorative study across three European countries. *PLoS One, 10*, e0129916.

Jonsson, L. S., Palmer, K., Ohlsson, H., Sundquist, J., & Sundquist, K. (2013). Is acculturation associated with physical activity among female immigrants in Sweden? *Journal of Public Health, 35*, 270–277.

Lara, M., Gamboa, C., Kahramanian, M. I., Morales, L. S., & Hayes-Bautista, D. E. (2005). Acculturation and Latino health in the United States: A review of the literature and its sociopolitical context. *Annual Review of Public Health, 26*, 367–397.

Loi, S., Rusciani, R., Spadea, T., Costa, G., & Egidi, V. (2018). Salute, stili di vita e accesso ai servizi sanitari [Health, lifestyles and access to health services]. In M. Perez et al. (Eds.), *Vita e integrazione sociale degli immigrati in Italia. [Life and social integration of immigrants in Italy]*. Rome: Istat.

Malmusi, D., Borrell, C., & Benach, J. (2010). Migration-related health inequalities: Showing the complex interactions between gender, social class and place of origin. *Social Science & Medicine, 71*, 1610–1619.

Maqoud, F., Vacca, E., & Tommaseo-Ponzetta, M. (2016). From Morocco to Italy: How women's bodies reflect their change of residence. *Collegium Antropologicum, 40*, 9–15.

Marin-Guerrero, A. C., Rodriguez-Artalejo, F., Guallar-Castillon, P., Lopez-Garcia, E., & Gutierrez-Fisac, J. L. (2015). Association of the duration of residence with obesity-related eating habits and dietary patterns among Latin-American immigrants in Spain. *The British Journal of Nutrition, 113*, 343–349.

McKay, L., MacIntyre, S., & Ellaway, A. (2003). *Migration and health: A review of the international literature*. Glasgow: MRC Social and Public Health Sciences Unit.

Mejean, C., Traissac, P., Eymard-Duvernay, S., El Ati, J., Delpeuch, F., & Maire, B. (2007). Influence of socio-economic and lifestyle factors on overweight and nutrition-related diseases among Tunisian migrants versus non-migrant Tunisians and French. *BMC Public Health, 7*, 265.

Nazroo, J. Y. (2003). The structuring of ethnic inequalities in health: Economic position, racial discrimination, and racism. *American Journal of Public Health, 93*, 277–284.

Pfarrwaller, E., & Suris, J. C. (2012). Determinants of health in recently arrived young migrants and refugees: A review of the literature. *Italian Journal of Public Health, 9*, e7529–e1–13.

Raberg Kjollesdal, M. K., Telle Hjellset, V., Bjorge, B., Holmboe-Ottesen, G., & Wandel, M. (2010). Barriers to healthy eating among Norwegian-Pakistani women participating in a culturally adapted intervention. *Scandinavian Journal of Public Health, 38*, 52–59.

Razum, O., Zeeb, H., & Rohrmann, S. (2000). The 'healthy migrant effect' – Not merely a fallacy of innacurate denominator figures. *International Journal of Epidemiology, 29*, 191–192.

Razum, O. (2006). Commentary: Of salmon and time travellers – Musing on the mystery of migrant mortality. *International Journal of Epidemiology, 35*, 919–921.

Robjant, K., Hassan, R., & Katona, C. (2009). Mental health implications of detaining asylum seekers: Systematic review. *The British Journal of Psychiatry, 194*, 306–312.

Rostila, M. (2010). Birds of a feather flock together – and fall ill? Migrant homophily and health in Sweden. *Sociology of Health & Illness, 32*, 382–399.

Scheppers, E., Van Dongen, E., Dekker, J., Geertzen, J. E., & Dekker, J. (2006). Potential barriers to the use of health services among ethnic minorities: A review. *Family Practice, 23*, 325–348.

Siddiqui, F., Lindblad, U., & Bennet, L. (2014). Physical inactivity is strongly associated with anxiety and depression in Iraqi immigrants to Sweden: A cross-sectional study. *BMC Public Health, 14*, 502.

Singh, M., & Kirchengast, S. (2011). Obesity prevalence and nutritional habits among Indian women: A comparison between Punjabi women living in India and Punjabi migrants in Vienna, Austria. *Anthropologischer Anzeiger, 68*, 239–251.

Spallek, J., Zeeb, H., & Razum, O. (2011). What do we have to know from migrants' past exposures to understand their health status? A life course approach. *Emerging Themes in Epidemiology, 8*, 6.

Ulmann, S. H., Goldman, N., & Massey, D. S. (2011). Healthier before they migrate, less healthy when they return? The health of returned migrants in Mexico. *Social Science & Medicine, 73*, 421–428.

Van Cleemput, P., Parry, G., Thomas, K., Peters, J., & Cooper, C. (2007). Health-related beliefs and experiences of gypsies and Travellers: A qualitative study. *Journal of Epidemiology & Community Health, 61*, 205–210.

Part II
Primary Health Care and Migrants: Quality, Adaptation, Best Practice and Health Policies

Chapter 7
Avoidable Hospitalization Among Migrants and Ethnic Minorities in Developed Economies

Laura Cacciani, Nera Agabiti, Marina Davoli, Teresa Dalla Zuanna, and Cristina Canova

7.1 Introduction

Global migration is increasing, especially labour migration of people moving from low income countries toward developed economies looking for work opportunities (UN 2015).

Entitlement to comprehensive use of healthcare services may depend on the legal status of migrants and on legislation in force in the host country. In addition, even when health systems include health assistance to migrants, formal or informal barriers may limit the accessibility of services (Norredam et al. 2010), and migrants may be often at risk of low quality of care.

Conditions for which hospitalization can be considered avoidable, through timely and effective preventive care and early disease management, are often referred to as ambulatory care sensitive conditions (ACSCs). The negative association between indicators of primary health care (PHC) accessibility and hospitalization for ACSCs (avoidable hospitalization, AH) has been reported in different studies showing lower AH rates in areas with greater access to PHC (Rosano et al. 2013).

Given the vulnerability of migrant populations to low quality of care, our purpose is to review and discuss the literature available on migrant status and AH in developed economies (as defined according to the country classification of the United Nations, UN) (UN 2016), taking into account the main differences among health systems and patterns of migration flows that may generate different patterns

L. Cacciani (✉) · N. Agabiti · M. Davoli
Department of Epidemiology of the Lazio Regional Health Service, ASL Roma 1, Rome, Italy
e-mail: l.cacciani@deplazio.it

T. D. Zuanna · C. Canova
Department of Cardiologic, Vascular and Thoracic Sciences, University of Padua, Padua, Italy

© The Author(s), under exclusive licence to Springer International Publishing AG, part of Springer Nature 2018
A. Rosano (ed.), *Access to Primary Care and Preventative Health Services of Migrants*, SpringerBriefs in Public Health, https://doi.org/10.1007/978-3-319-73630-3_7

67

of AH, and to discuss the use of AH as a proxy of quality of primary care in this context. Therefore, we will summarize the characteristics of the principal health systems and healthcare assistance in developed economies, the main characteristics of migration flows and health-related issues, the concepts and definitions for AH, discussing its use as an indicator of quality of care. Then we will discuss the available data sources useful to produce evidence on migrant status and AH, and we will review the available scientific literature. We will consider international migration, in particular toward European countries, while we will not focus on forced migration.

7.2   Main Health Systems and Healthcare Assistance Models in Developed Economies

The interpretation of health indicators with respect to migrant status or ethnicity may change in relation to the scheme of health coverage in force in each country, which may or not include payment in charge of migrants, especially for unemployed, irregular or undocumented migrants. While the health system of the United States is mainly based on private insurance and out-of-pocket payments, those of most developed economies rely on social health insurance (some European countries and Japan) or tax-financed systems (some other European countries, Australia, Canada, New Zealand). Health systems so different may impact on health outcomes (Wagstaff 2009), and as a consequence may generate health differentials between migrant and non-migrant populations due to health coverage disparities and entitlement to benefit from available healthcare services. In addition, many other different potential barriers may impact on the access to healthcare services among migrants and ethnic minorities. According to a review on this issue, such barriers may occur at patient level, provider level and system level, and depend on the particular situation of the individual patient (Scheppers et al. 2006).

7.3   Migration Flows in Developed Economies and Health-Related Issues

In 2015, the number of international migrants, that is, according to the UN, people residing in a country other than their either country of birth or citizenship, reached about 244 million people in the world, with an increase of about 41% since 2000. Most of them are of working ages and nearly 58% lived in developed regions such as United States (47.6 million), Germany (12.0), United Kingdom (8.5), Canada and France (7.8 each), Australia (6.7) and Spain (5.8) (UN 2015). According to Eurostat, the number of people residing in an EU member State with citizenship of a non-member country was 20.7 million in 2016, representing 4.1% of the EU-28 population. In addition, there were 16.0 million persons living in one of the EU member States with the citizenship of another EU member State (Eurostat 2017).

The health status of migrants is heterogeneous across developed economies, depending on multiple factors related to origin and hosting countries, and to the migratory history and experience of migrants as individuals or as groups. Although it is difficult to summarize the health status of migrants (Rechel et al. 2011), the available evidence shows that health problems of migrants in different settings and places have been found to be related to maternal and child health (Almeida et al. 2013), perinatal outcomes (Urquia et al. 2010; Cacciani et al. 2011), diabetes (Montesi et al. 2016), some infectious diseases (European Observatory on Health Systems and Policies 2014; William and Noori 2014), occupational health and injuries (Ahonen et al. 2007; Salvatore et al. 2013), and mental health (Kirmayer et al. 2011).

Concerning most recent large scale migration due to the economic downturn and political instability in the area of North Africa and the Middle East, the key health problems affecting migrants include accidental injuries, hypothermia, burns, gastrointestinal illnesses, cardiovascular events, pregnancy- and delivery-related complications, diabetes and hypertension (WHO Europe 2017).

Access to healthcare is an issue for migrant populations, even in countries where legal entitlements are guaranteed to them (Rechel et al. 2013), and systematic variations in healthcare services utilization between migrants and non-migrants have been observed (Norredam et al. 2010). As a consequence, quality of care to migrant may be questionable and their health status may deteriorate.

7.4 AH: Concepts and Definitions, Its Use as an Indicator of Quality of Care

7.4.1 Definition and General Meaning

Ambulatory Care Sensitive Conditions (ACSCs) are a subset of diseases where hospital admission is potentially avoidable by preventing the onset of disease (e.g. influenza vaccination), controlling an acute episodic illness (e.g. dehydration and gastroenteritis), or managing a chronic condition effectively (e.g. complications of diabetes) (Gibson et al. 2013; Means 2016; Yam et al. 2010). Since ACSCs are considered avoidable by appropriate and timely outpatient care, hospitalization for ACSCs is frequently named unnecessary or avoidable hospitalization (AH). Disease prevention and monitoring chronic conditions are key points at the primary care level, then hospitalization for ACSCs is frequently used as a quality indicator for primary care settings (Van Loenen et al. 2016; Cecil et al. 2015; Rosano et al. 2013). The concept of AH originated in New York in the early 1990s and since then has been widely used as an indicator of effectiveness of, or access to, primary healthcare in many countries (Cecil et al. 2015; AHRQ 2001; OECD 2015). The relationship between better access to primary care and fewer admissions for ACSCs has been shown in several studies (Gibson et al. 2013; Van Loenen et al. 2016; Busby et al. 2015). Moreover, the impact on health care resources and expenditures related to AH has been documented worldwide as large and alarming (Busby et al. 2017b, Weeks et al. 2016). Compared with patients without ACSCs admission, a larger proportion of patients with ACSCs hospitalization required advanced treatment or died on admission (Mkanta et al. 2016).

While examining the large body of literature on ACSCs and AH, a wide range of different types and definitions of ACSCs to be included is evident (Van Loenen et al. 2016; Busby et al. 2015). This is the reason why it is difficult to summarize results and conclusions from studies in different countries. Diabetes and related complications, Angina, Chronic Obstructive Pulmonary Disease (COPD), Congestive Heart Failure (CHF) in adult and elderly population are the most important ACSCs and are included in the majority of studies, while Gastroenteritis and Pneumonia account for AH in children (Gibson et al. 2013; Means et al. 2016; Yam et al. 2010; Cecil et al. 2015). Hospital admissions for patients with Diabetes, CHF, COPD, and Asthma are routinely reported within EU countries' health system performance frameworks as part of their healthcare quality assessment (Calderón-Larrañaga et al. 2011; P.Re.Val.E 2017). They are also routinely used as indicators of the performance of primary care systems by the Organization for Economic Co-operation and Development (OECD 2015). Finally, AH rates have been widely used to quantify inequity in care delivery for populations with socioeconomic disadvantages or more vulnerable in comparison to their well-off counterparts (Khanassov et al. 2016; McCormick et al. 2015; Johnson et al. 2012).

7.4.2   Relationship Between Primary Care and AH

It has been hypothesized that healthcare systems with easy access to primary care have lower hospitalization rates because problems are detected at an earlier stage and disease deterioration can be prevented. A large body of evidence confirm this hypothesis (Gibson et al. 2013; Means et al. 2016; Yam et al. 2010). However, the mechanisms are complex and the strong relationship between quality of primary care and AH has been recently questioned (Gibson et al. 2013; Walker et al. 2017; Falster et al. 2015). A complete understanding of the causes of AH is difficult and requires examination of many aspects, both at individual and at contextual level (Busby et al. 2015, 2017a; Hong and Kang 2013). While aging populations are common in many countries, differences in organization and delivery of care to tackle with their complex health needs may influence the type and the number of AH and lead to different interpretation and usefulness of this quality indicator in each country (van Loenen et al. 2014; Delamater et al. 2013). A number of observational studies examines single causes of AH instead of a large list of ACSCs (Van Loenen et al. 2016; Calderón-Larrañaga et al. 2011). Particular attention has been paid to hospitalization for diabetes and diabetes-related conditions. Several studies have shown that patients with a continuous relationship with their primary care provider have less chance of being admitted for diabetes complications; in particular, patients treated by multidisciplinary teams have fewer hospital admissions (Gibson et al. 2013; Rosano et al. 2013; Manns et al. 2012). In contrast, it has been shown that where primary care practices have more medical equipment and high task profile physicians, rates of hospital admission for uncontrolled diabetes tend to be higher (Van Loenen et al. 2016). In some countries, lower rates of AH were found in urban areas, this was not the case in rural areas suggesting that contextual factors, individual socioeconomic and behavioural factors and healthcare characteristics may interact in determining AH rates (Falster et al. 2015; Delamater et al. 2013). In general, the main limitation of this indicator is the fact that the proportion of AH that is actually preventable is unknown and there is no easy way for a health system or researchers to identify which individual admissions are actually preventable (Passey et al. 2015). Another critical point consists in the fact that ACSCs are frequently identified on the basis of diagnostic codes in hospital administrative data. While this approach takes advantage of the availability of administrative datasets, it may overestimate rates of preventable admissions because it also captures an unknown number of admissions that are necessary and could not feasibly have been prevented (Walker et al. 2017; Passey et al. 2015; Sundmacher et al. 2015). More recently, emergency visits for ACSCs have been also suggested as a proxy of inadequate primary care (Johnson et al. 2012).

7.4.3 Geographical Variability: Interpretation and Challenges

Updated international comparison of AH rates comes from a report by the OECD (OECD 2015). As regards diabetes, OECD indicates that in 2013 there were almost 7-fold variations in the admission rate for diabetes among countries across Europe. Age-adjusted admission rates for diabetes varied from 44 per 100,000 in Italy and Switzerland to 231 and 296 per 100,000 in Poland and Austria respectively. With the exception of Poland, Latvia and Slovenia, most countries have seen a reduction in diabetes admission rates over the past 5 years. Countries such as Italy, Finland and Switzerland saw a decline of more than 30% in admission rates for diabetes between 2007 and 2013. Variation in AH across areas in a single country or region has also been reported (Busby et al. 2015; P.Re.Val.E 2017). Primary care quality and secondary care access were frequently suggested as drivers of AH variation, however several different methods were used to quantify variation and comparison of results and conclusions across studies are difficult (Busby 2015). In the recent work from an international focus group on behalf of the European Commission (EC) it was noted that validation and interpretation of AH as indicator of quality of diabetes care vary across countries, as well as its utility and usage (European Commission Directorate General for Health and Food Safety 2016). Then, caution in interpreting international comparison is needed. Again, from the updated EC report it is clear that complex conditions require multi-sectoral and multidisciplinary approaches.

There is a need to develop new indicators to provide information on the coordination between sectors, in particular primary and secondary care. New approaches linking hospital registries data with other sources, such as disease registers, or using data on co-morbidities or multiple diagnoses may lead to a better understanding of the patient profile and of the quality of integrated care pathways for chronic conditions (Passey et al. 2015; European Commission Directorate General for Health and Food Safety 2016). Lastly, it has been suggested the need to disaggregate avoidable admissions and examine specific conditions, taking into account that indicator robustness varies for different diseases (European Commission Directorate General for Health and Food Safety 2016).

7.4.4   Issues Related to AH as an Indicator of Primary Care Among Migrants

The interpretation of AH as an indicator of quality of care, especially of primary care, may be even more challenging when comparing results across subgroups of populations, such as migrants and ethnic minorities. For example, it has been shown that migrants may be subject to a myriad of barriers when accessing primary care (Scheppers et al. 2006), which may be heterogeneous across ethnic groups and host countries. Again, AH may be not only driven by quality of primary and secondary care (Busby et al. 2015), but also by the inadequacy of health systems to meet the needs of migrant groups.

Any finding on differentials of AH across migrant and non-migrant populations should be therefore interpreted with caution and possibly in relation to individual and contextual adjustment variables.

7.5   Data Sources on Migrant Populations and Hospitalization

The concept of migrant is difficult to define, being measured with nationality, birthplace, ethnicity, or race as in the USA, and as a consequence it is difficult to find datasets including migrant-sensitive information comparable within and across countries. In addition, such information is sparse and not routinely collected in demographic or health statistics, hampering the chance to measure health related indicators (Rechel et al. 2013). However, in many developed economies demographic statistics are available, e.g. the census or municipal registers, and allow to identify citizenship or birthplace, and may provide denominators to calculate health indicators. Administrative data on hospitalization, which allow to calculate hospitalization rates numerators, are available so far in many European countries (Nielsen et al. 2009), and in the USA where many studies on avoidable hospitalization are based on the Healthcare Cost and Utilization Project (HCUP) which is the Nation's most comprehensive source of hospital care data (AHRQ 2017). Nevertheless, it is necessary to be aware of potential misclassification of migrants, and of bias and lack of generalizability due to migrants not included in the official statistics.

7.6   Literature Review on Migrant Status and AH

In June 2015, a systematic literature review was conducted to produce evidence on all the studies published to date on AH among ethnic minorities and migrant groups, in Europe and elsewhere (Dalla Zuanna et al. 2017). Studies presenting AH rates and/or rate ratios between at least two different ethnic groups or between migrants and natives were searched in primary electronic databases. This review identified 35 original articles, of whom 21 papers presented overall AH rates.

In order to provide a comprehensive review in this Chapter, the literature search has been updated up to June 2017, using the same search strategy and focusing only on the studies that presented overall AH rates among different ethnic groups and migrant groups. Nine recently published studied were retrieved (Chopra et al. 2016; Gonçalves et al. 2016; Hale et al. 2016; Heo et al. 2015; Lessard et al. 2016; Matheson et al. 2015; Mukamel et al. 2015; Potter et al. 2016; Wright et al. 2017), bringing to a total of 30 studies: 21 were conducted in the USA, five in New Zealand, two in Australia, one in Singapore and one in Brazil; none European study was identified. Most of the studies had a cross-sectional design (n = 26), analysed rates in the general population considering different age groups (n = 21). The terms "race", "ethnicity", or the two terms combined, were used as exposure variable in 29 studies. In the studies conducted in the United States, the terms used were often "White/Black race", with or without "Hispanic ethnicity", sometimes mentioning other ethnic minorities. In the studies conducted in New Zealand, Singapore and Brazil, the exposure variable was based on ethnicity. One Australian study considered indigenous and non-indigenous populations. The other Australian study was the only one considering country of birth as a proxy of migrant status, to compare Australian citizens with people coming from eight refugee-source countries. Twenty-five studies reported an adjustment for age and other covariates; of these, 13 included socioeconomic status or a proxy of it. As regards the outcome, all the studies assessed AH rates/rates ratio using hospital discharge records. Eleven studies applied the American Agency of Healthcare Research and Quality (AHRQ 2016) definition, while six studies adopted the list proposed by Billings. In the other studies the authors chose other published lists of ACSCs (6 studies), a list proposed for the national context (3 studies) or drew up their own list (2 studies).

Figure 7.1 shows the overall AH rates, stratified by exposure variable and setting. All the considered studies from the United States showed higher rates (up to 2.4 fold) for the Black race or African American ethnicity than their White/EU counterparts. Also Hispanics and other ethnic minorities had higher AH rates than

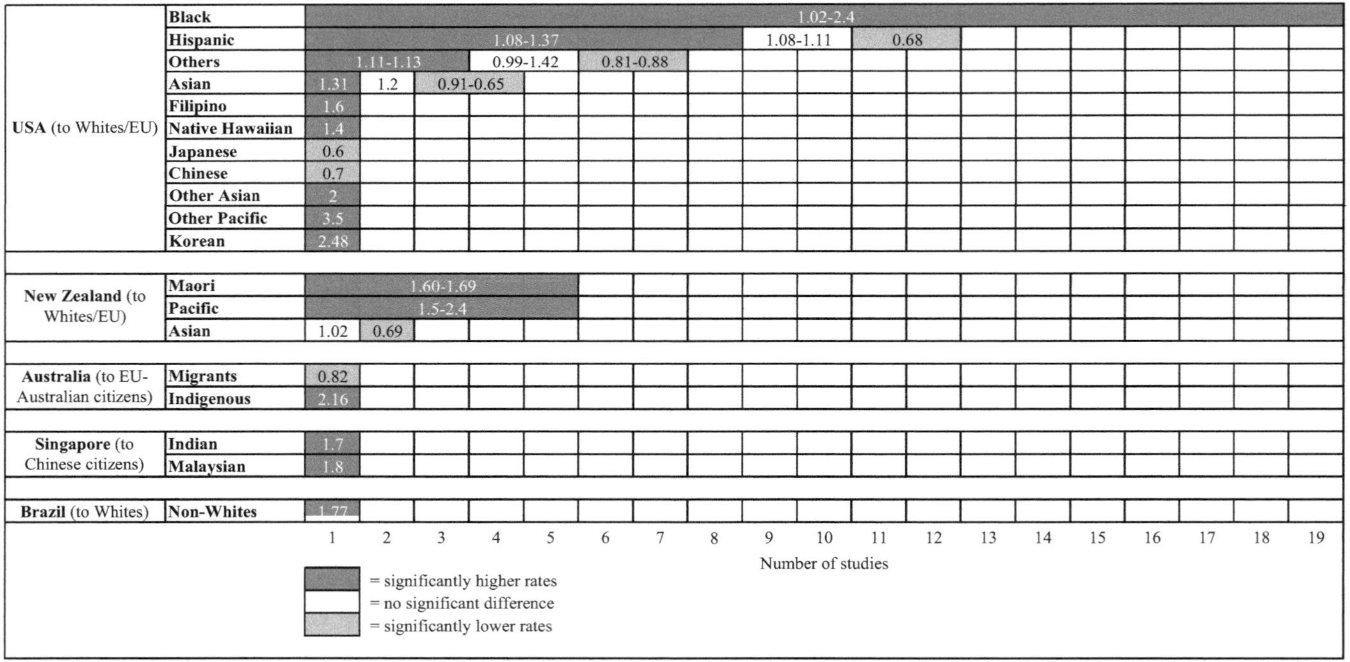

Fig. 7.1 Results of 30 studies presenting overall AH rates, showing the range of the rate ratios for each racial/ethnic group stratified by geographical setting

whites/EU. The Asian group and the Chinese and Japanese in Hawaii had largely similar or lower rates than the White/European group. In New Zealand, Singapore, Australia and Brazil, ethnic minorities had usually higher AH rates than the majority group. An exception to this is the Asian group in New Zealand who experienced rates lower than or similar to the latter, and migrants from refugee-source countries in the Australian study, where AH rates were lower for this group.

AH is an outcome measure of the performance of Primary Health Care, and it has been widely used, mainly in the recent years (9 out of the 30 included studies were published in the last 2 years) to underline disparities in primary healthcare performance among different racial/ethnic groups, especially in the USA. This updated review still underlined the lack of studies conducted in a European setting.

We focused only on the studies that used an overall measure of AH, because due to the specificity of our search strategy we had included only articles where the authors specifically described the conditions included in the list of ACSCs as "avoidable". That is the reason why we conducted additional searches focusing on asthma and diabetes, trying to identify European studies.

7.6.1   Hospitalization for Asthma and Diabetes Among Migrants

Numerous studies, mainly set in the USA, have documented racial disparities in asthma management and outcomes, among which asthma hospitalizations in children and young adults that are potentially avoidable through regular ambulatory care by specialty and primary care physicians. In particular, black children, and to a lesser extent black adults, have been shown to have up to three times increased hospitalization rates compared with white patients (Akinbami et al. 2014; Moorman et al. 2012; Getahun et al. 2005). The underlying causes of these disparities include inadequate access to healthcare, lower socioeconomic status, suboptimal use of asthma controller medications, environmental exposures, genetic and behavioural differences, and healthcare provider shortcomings (e.g. poor communication or racial bias) (Erickson et al. 2007).

Therefore, a systematic review of studies conducted in Europe on asthma hospitalization among ethnic minorities and migrant groups has been conducted in June/July 2017. Only few UK (Netuveli et al. 2005; Sheikh et al. 2016) and Sweden studies were identified (Hjern et al. 1999; Li et al. 2013a). In line with previous studies from USA, a UK systematic review found that south Asians and black children and young adults were at significantly increased risk of admission for asthma (Netuveli et al. 2005). A recent population-based cohort study in the Scottish population (without age restriction) showed that compared to the reference White Scottish population, people of South Asian descent (i.e. Pakistani, Indian and Other South Asians) had 20–50% increased rates of hospitalization from asthma, whereas people of Chinese origin had 30–40% lower rates, and people with African origin experienced similar rates (Sheikh et al. 2016). On the contrary, the two studies conducted in Sweden found a lower risk of asthma-related hospitalization among children born outside Sweden (Hjern et al. 1999) and among children born to immigrant mothers (Li et al. 2013a).

Many studies, again mainly from the USA, have highlighted ethnic differences also in hospitalization rates for type 2 diabetes, with Blacks, Hispanics and other ethnic minorities often presenting higher rates compared to their white counterpart (Khan et al.2011; Sentell et al. 2013; Fisher and Ma 2015). The observed disparity may be partially explained by different prevalence of the disease, as epidemiological studies have shown that the prevalence of type 2 diabetes may vary markedly across ethnic groups (Wild et al. 2004; Forouhi et al. 2005; Shamshirgaran et al. 2013). Diabetes is a multifactorial disease (Doria et al. 2008), and both genetic and environmental factors (e.g. obesity, sedentary lifestyle, stress, nutritional factors) are differently distributed across ethnic groups. Differences in admission rates may also be linked to socioeconomic disadvantage (Li et al. 2013b), or to different health-seeking behaviour or primary care management (Nuti et al. 2012).

A systematic review of the literature has been conducted in July 2017 in order to search for studies set in Europe comparing hospitalization for type 2 diabetes among adults in different ethnic or migrant groups. The search identified one Sweden study (Li et al. 2013b) and one from the UK (Nishino et al. 2015). In the Sweden study, hospitalization rates were analysed both for first and second generation of immigrants. Findings for the first generation were mixed, with sometimes higher and sometimes lower rates, considering each country of origin (or area) separately, and a slightly increased overall risk. Increased or decreased risks disappeared in most of the second-generation immigrants (Li et al. 2013b). These finding may suggest that environmental factors may be important to explain the observed variation in hospitalization for diabetes, and that access barriers to PHC might be lower for the second generation of immigrants. The study from UK found that ethnic minority groups (particularly south Asians) were at higher risk of hospital admission for diabetes compared to white British people, but these differences disappeared when considering the readmission rate (Nishino et al. 2015). These finding may be explained by higher prevalence of type 2 diabetes and care in some ethnic groups that may have improved the diabetic condition.

Although ethnic minority and migrant populations are considered vulnerable healthcare groups, research on asthma and diabetes avoidable hospitalization is lacking in the European context and this warrants further research because of the possible implications for disease prevention.

7.7 Conclusions and Perspectives

Definitions, concepts, and scientific literature related to migration, health, and AH as an indicator of quality of primary care, in different developed economies with different health systems, have been presented and discussed, and the main factors hampering comparisons within and across studies and countries have been described. The important dimension of international migration has been also described, and the lack of European studies on migration and AH has been documented through the literature review.

Available evidence often shows overall higher AH among migrants compared to non-migrants. This result may indicate a susceptibility of migrants to low quality of primary care in developed economies, though a variability of results has been observed. Heterogeneity may depend on many factors, some uncontrolled, such as ethnicity, socioeconomic position, age and aging, comorbidity, study population, country, setting, group of diseases or single disease investigated, prevalence of diseases, study design and exposure measurements.

There is a need for additional research to produce further evidence in order to assess and then avoid human and economic costs of inefficiencies in primary care, taking into account previous experience on study design, methodology and issues related to migrants' health.

Acknowledgements We wish to thank Andrea Bardin (Resident Physician, Postgraduate School of Hygiene and Preventive Medicine, University of Padua, Italy) for his contribution to the review of the most recent literature about AH among migrants.

References

AHRQ Quality Indicators—Guide to Prevention Quality Indicators: Hospital Admission for Ambulatory Care Sensitive Conditions. Rockville, MD: Agency for Healthcare Research and Quality, 2001. AHRQ Pub. No. 02-R0203. https://www.ahrq.gov/downloads/pub/ahrqqi/pqi-guide.pdf. Accessed 3 July 2017.

Agency for Healthcare Research and Quality (AHRQ). (2017). Healthcare Cost and Utilization Project (HCUP). https://www.ahrq.gov/research/data/hcup/index.html. Accessed 3 July 2017.

Agency for Healthcare Research and Quality (AHRQ). (2016, October). Prevention Quality Indicators Technical Specifications Updates – Version 6.0 (ICD-9). https://www.qualityindicators.ahrq.gov/Modules/PQI_TechSpec_ICD09_v60.aspx. Accessed 24 June 2017.

Ahonen, E. Q., Benavides, F. G., & Benach, J. (2007). Immigrant populations, work and health-a systematic literature review. *Scandinavian Journal of Work, Environment & Health, 33*(2), 96–104.

Akinbami, L. J., Moorman, J. E., Simon, A. E., & Schoendorf, K. C. (2014). Trends in racial disparities for asthma outcomes among children 0 to 17 years, 2001–2010. *The Journal of Allergy and Clinical Immunology, 134*(3), 547–553. e5.

Almeida, L. M., Caldas, J., Ayres-de-Campos, D., Salcedo-Barrientos, D., & Dias, S. (2013). Maternal healthcare in migrants: A systematic review. *Maternal and Child Health Journal, 17*, 1346–1354. https://doi.org/10.1007/s10995-012-1149-x.

Busby, J., Purdy, S., & Hollingworth, W. (2015). A systematic review of the magnitude and cause of geographic variation in unplanned hospital admission rates and length of stay for ambulatory care sensitive conditions. *BMC Health Services Research, 15*, 324. https://doi.org/10.1186/s12913-015-0964-3.

Busby, J., Purdy, S., & Hollingworth, W. (2017a). How do population, general practice and hospital factors influence ambulatory care sensitive admissions: A cross sectional study. *BMC Family Practice, 18*, 67. https://doi.org/10.1186/s12875-017-0638-9.

Busby, J., Purdy, S., & Hollingworth, W. (2017b). Using geographic variation in unplanned ambulatory care sensitive condition admission rates to identify commissioning priorities: An analysis of routine data from England. *Journal of Health Services Research & Policy, 22*, 20–27. https://doi.org/10.1177/1355819616666397.

Cacciani, L., Asole, S., Polo, A., Franco, F., Lucchini, R., De Curtis, M., et al. (2011). Perinatal outcomes among immigrant mothers over two periods in a region of central Italy. *BMC Public Health, 11*, 294. https://doi.org/10.1186/1471-2458-11-294.

Calderón-Larrañaga, A., Carney, L., Soljak, M., Bottle, A., Partridge, M., Bell, D., et al. (2011). Association of population and primary healthcare factors with hospital admission rates for chronic obstructive pulmonary disease in England: National cross-sectional study. *Thorax, 66*, 191–196. https://doi.org/10.1136/thx.2010.147058.

Cecil, E., Bottle, A., Sharland, M., & Saxena, S. (2015). Impact of UK primary care policy reforms on short-stay unplanned hospital admissions for children with primary care-sensitive conditions. *Annals of Family Medicine, 13*, 214–220. https://doi.org/10.1370/afm.1786.

Chopra, I., Wilkins, T. L., & Sambamoorthi, U. (2016). Ambulatory care sensitive hospitalizations among Medicaid beneficiaries with chronic conditions. *Hospital Practice (1995)., 44*, 48–59. https://doi.org/10.1080/21548331.2016.1144446.

Dalla Zuanna, T., Spadea, T., Milana, M., Petrelli, A., Cacciani, L., Simonato, L., et al. (2017). Avoidable hospitalisation among migrants and ethnic minority groups: A systematic review. *European Journal of Public Health, 27*(5), 861–868.

Delamater, P. L., Messina, J. P., Grady, S. C., et al. (2013). Do more hospital beds lead to higher hospitalization rates? A spatial examination of Roemer's Law. *PLoS One, 8*, e54900. https://doi.org/10.1371/journal.pone.0054900.

Doria A, Patti ME, Kahn CR. The emerging genetic architecture of type 2 diabetes. Cell Metab. 2008;8:186–200. doi:10.1016/j.cmet.2008.08.006.

Erickson, S. E., Iribarren, C., Tolstykh, I. V., Blanc, P. D., & Eisner, M. D. (2007). Effect of race on asthma management and outcomes in a large, integrated managed care organization. *Archives of Internal Medicine, 167*(17), 1846–1852.

European Commission Directorate General for Health and Food Safety. (2016). So what? Strategies across Europe to assess quality of care. Report by the Expert Group on Health Systems Performance Assessment. https://ec.europa.eu/health//sites/health/files/systems_performance_assessment/docs/sowhat_en.pdf. Accessed 24 July 2017.

European Observatory on Health Systems and Policies: Migrants and health. (2014). http://www.euro.who.int/__data/assets/pdf_file/0011/266186/Eurohealth-v20-n4_1.pdf?ua=1. Accessed 3 July 2017.

Eurostat. (2017). Migration and migrant population statistics. http://ec.europa.eu/eurostat/statistics-explained/index.php/Migration_and_migrant_population_statistics#Migration_flows. Accessed 3 July 2017.

Falster, M. O., Jorm, L. R., Douglas, K. A., et al. (2015). Sociodemographic and health characteristics, rather than primary care supply, are major drivers of geographic variation in preventable hospitalizations in Australia. *Medical Care, 53*, 436–445. https://doi.org/10.1097/MLR.0000000000000342.

Fisher, M. A., & Ma, Z. Q. (2015). Medicaid-insured and uninsured were more likely to have diabetes emergency/urgent admissions. *The American Journal of Managed Care, 21*(5), e312–e319.

Forouhi, N. G., Merrick, D., Goyder, E., Ferguson, B. A., Abbas, J., Lachowycz, K., & Wild, S. H. (2005). Diabetes prevalence in England, 2001—estimates from an epidemiological model. *Diabetic Medicine, 23*, 189–197.

Getahun, D., Demissie, K., & Rhoads, G. G. (2005). Recent trends in asthma hospitalization and mortality in the United States. *The Journal of Asthma, 42*(5), 373–378.

Gibson, O. R., Segal, L., & McDermott, R. A. (2013). A systematic review of evidence on the association between hospitalisation for chronic disease related ambulatory care sensitive conditions and primary health care resourcing. *BMC Health Services Research, 13*, 336. https://doi.org/10.1186/1472-6963-13-336.

Gonçalves, M. R., Hauser, L., Prestes, I. V., Schmidt, M. I., Duncan, B. B., & Harzheim, E. (2016). Primary health care quality and hospitalizations for ambulatory care sensitive conditions in the public health system in Porto Alegre, Brazil. *Family Practice, 33*, 238–242. https://doi.org/10.1093/fampra/cmv051.

Hale, N., Probst, J., & Robertson, A. (2016). Rural area deprivation and hospitalizations among children for ambulatory care sensitive conditions. *Journal of Community Health, 41*, 451–460. https://doi.org/10.1007/s10900-015-0113-2.

Heo, H. H., Sentell, T. L., Li, D., Ahn, H. J., Miyamura, J., & Braun, K. (2015). Disparities in potentially preventable hospitalizations for chronic conditions among Korean Americans, Hawaii, 2010–2012. *Preventing Chronic Disease, 12*, E152. https://doi.org/10.5888/pcd12.150057.

Hjern, A., Haglund, B., Bremberg, S., & Ringbäck-Weitoft, G. (1999). Social adversity, migration and hospital admissions for childhood asthma in Sweden. *Acta Paediatrica, 88*(10), 1107–1112.

Hong, J. S., & Kang, H. C. (2013). Continuity of ambulatory care and health outcomes in adult patients with type 2 diabetes in Korea. *Health Policy, 109*, 158–165. https://doi.org/10.1016/j.healthpol.2012.09.009.

Johnson, P. J., Ghildayal, N., Ward, A. C., Westgard, B. C., Boland, L. L., & Hokanson, J. S. (2012). Disparities in potentially avoidable emergency department (ED) care: ED visits for ambulatory care sensitive conditions. *Medical Care, 50*, 1020–1028. https://doi.org/10.1097/MLR.0b013e318270bad4.

Khan, N. A., Wang, H., Anand, S., Jin, Y., Campbell, N., Pilote, L., et al. (2011). Ethnicity and sex affect diabetes incidence and outcome. *Diabetes Care, 34*, 96–101.

Khanassov, V., Pluye, P., Descoteaux, S., Haggerty, J. L., Russell, G., Gunn, J., et al. (2016). Organizational interventions improving access to community-based primary health care for vulnerable populations: A scoping review. *International Journal for Equity in Health, 15*(1), 168.

Kirmayer, L. J., Narasiah, L., Munoz, M., Rashid, M., Ryder, A. G., Guzder, J., et al. (2011). Common mental health problems in immigrants and refugees: General approach in primary care. *CMAJ, 183*, E959–E967. https://doi.org/10.1503/cmaj.090292.

Lessard, L. N., Alcala, E., & Capitman, J. A. (2016). Pollution, poverty, and potentially preventable childhood morbidity in Central California. *The Journal of Pediatrics, 168*, 198–204. https://doi.org/10.1016/j.jpeds.2015.08.007.

Li, X., Sundquist, J., Calling, S., Zöller, B., & Sundquist, K. (2013a). Mothers, places and risk of hospitalization for childhood asthma: A nationwide study from Sweden: Epidemiology of allergic disease. *Clinical and Experimental Allergy, 43*(6), 652–658.

Li, X., Sundquist, J., Zöller, B., Bennet, L., & Sundquist, K. (2013b). Risk of hospitalization for type 2 diabetes in first- and second-generation immigrants in Sweden: A nationwide follow-up study. *Journal of Diabetes and its Complications, 27*(1), 49–45.

Manns, B. J., Tonelli, M., Zhang, J., et al. (2012). Enrolment in primary care networks: Impact on outcomes and processes of care for patients with diabetes. *CMAJ, 184*, E144–E152. https://doi.org/10.1503/cmaj.110755.

Matheson, D., Reidy, J., Tan, L., & Carr, J. (2015). Good progress for children coupled with recalcitrant inequalities for adults in New Zealand's journey towards universal health coverage over the last decade. *The New Zealand Medical Journal, 128*(1415), 14–24.

McCormick, D., Hanchate, A. D., Lasser, K. E., Manze, M. G., Lin, M., Chu, C., et al. (2015). Effect of Massachusetts healthcare reform on racial and ethnic disparities in admissions to hospital for ambulatory care sensitive conditions: Retrospective analysis of hospital episode statistics. *BMJ, 350*, h1480. https://doi.org/10.1136/bmj.h1480.

Means, T. (2016). Improving quality of care and reducing unnecessary hospital admissions: A literature review. *British Journal of Community Nursing, 21*, 288–291. https://doi.org/10.12968/bjcn.2016.21.6.284.

Mkanta, W. N., Chumbler, N. R., Yang, K., Saigal, R., & Abdollahi, M. (2016). Cost and predictors of hospitalizations for ambulatory care - sensitive conditions among Medicaid enrollees in comprehensive managed care plans. *Health Services Research and Managerial Epidemiology, 3*, 2333392816670301. https://doi.org/10.1177/2333392816670301.

Montesi, L., Caletti, M. T., & Marchesini, G. (2016). Diabetes in migrants and ethnic minorities in a changing world. *World Journal of Diabetes, 7*, 34–44. https://doi.org/10.4239/wjd.v7.i3.34.

Moorman, J. E., Akinbami, L. J., Bailey, C. M., Zahran, H. S., King, M. E., Johnson, C. A., & Liu, X. (2012). National surveillance of asthma: United States, 2001-2010. *Vital & Health Statistics. Series 3, Analytical and Epidemiological Studies, 35*, 1–58.

Mukamel, D. B., Ladd, H., Li, Y., Temkin-Greener, H., & Ngo-Metzger, Q. (2015). Have racial disparities in ambulatory care sensitive admissions abated over time? *Medical Care, 53*, 931–939. https://doi.org/10.1097/MLR.0000000000000426.

Netuveli, G., Hurwitz, B., & Sheikh, A. (2005). Ethnic variations in incidence of asthma episodes in England & Wales: National study of 502,482 patients in primary care. *Respiratory Research, 6*, 120.

Nielsen, S., Krasnik, A., & Rosano, A. (2009). Registry data for cross-country comparisons of migrants' healthcare utilization in the EU: A survey study of availability and content. *BMC Health Services Research, 9*, 210. https://doi.org/10.1186/1472-6963-9-210.

Nishino, Y., Gilmour, S., & Shibuya, K. (2015). Inequality in diabetes-related hospital admissions in England by socioeconomic deprivation and ethnicity: Facility-based cross-sectional analysis. *PLoS One, 10*(2), e0116689.

Norredam, M., Nielsen, S. S., & Krasnik, A. (2010). Migrants' utilization of somatic healthcare services in Europe--a systematic review. *European Journal of Public Health, 20*, 555–563. https://doi.org/10.1093/eurpub/ckp195.

Nuti, L. A., Lawley, M., Turkcan, A., Tian, Z., Zhang, L., Chang, K., Willis, D. R., & Sands, L. P. (2012). No-shows to primary care appointments: Subsequent acute care utilization among diabetic patients. *BMC Health Services Research, 12*, 304.

OECD Health Care Quality Indicator project. (2015, Revision). http://www.oecd.org/els/health-systems/health-care-quality-indicators.htm. Accessed 24 July 2017.

P.Re.Val.E. (2017, Edition). Regional Program Outcomes Evaluation Lazio Region. http://95.110.213.190/prevale2017/index.php. Accessed 24 July 2017.

Passey, M. E., Longman, J. M., Johnston, J. J., Jorm, L., Ewald, D., Morgan, G. G., et al. (2015). Diagnosing Potentially Preventable Hospitalisations (DaPPHne): Protocol for a mixed-methods data-linkage study. *BMJ Open, 5*, e009879. https://doi.org/10.1136/bmjopen-2015-009879.

Potter, A. J., Trivedi, A. N., & Wright, B. (2016). Younger dual-Eligibles who use federally qualified health centers have more preventable emergency department visits, but some have fewer hospitalizations. *Journal of Primary Care & Community Health, 8*(1), 3–8.

Rechel, B., Mladovsky, P., Devillé, W., Rijks, B., Petrova-Benedict, R., & McKee, M. (2011). Migration and health in the European Union: An introduction. In B. Rechel, P. Mladovsky, W. Devillé, B. Rijks, R. Petrova-Benedict, & M. McKee (Eds.), *Migration and health in the European Union* (pp. 3–13). Maidenhead: Open University Press.

Rechel, B., Mladovsky, P., Ingleby, D., Mackenbach, J. P., & McKee, M. (2013). Migration and health in an increasingly diverse Europe. *Lancet, 381*, 1235–1245. https://doi.org/10.1016/S0140-6736(12)62086-8.

Rosano, A., Loha, C. A., Falvo, R., van der Zee, J., Ricciardi, W., Guasticchi, G., et al. (2013). The relationship between avoidable hospitalization and accessibility to primary care: A systematic review. *European Journal of Public Health, 23*, 356–360. https://doi.org/10.1093/eurpub/cks053.

Salvatore, M. A., Baglio, G., Cacciani, L., Spagnolo, A., & Rosano, A. (2013). Work-related injuries among immigrant workers in Italy. *Journal of Immigrant and Minority Health, 15*, 182–187. https://doi.org/10.1007/s10903-012-9673-8.

Scheppers, E., van Dongen, E., Dekker, J., Geertzen, J., & Dekker, J. (2006). Potential barriers to the use of health services among ethnic minorities: A review. *Family Practice, 23*(3), 325–348.

Sentell, T. L., Ahn, H. J., Juarez, D. T., Tseng, C., Chen, J. J., Salvail, F. L., et al. (2013). Comparison of potentially preventable hospitalizations related to diabetes among native Hawaiian, Chinese,

Filipino and Japanese elderly compared with Whites, Hawai'i, December 2006-December 2010. *Preventing Chronic Disease, 10*, 120340.

Shamshirgaran, S. M., Jorm, L., Bambrick, H., & Hennessy, A. (2013). Independent roles of country of birth and socioeconomic status in the occurrence of type 2 diabetes. *BMC Public Health, 13*, 1223.

Sheikh, A., Steiner, M. F., Cezard, G., Bansal, N., Fischbacher, C., Simpson, C. R., Douglas, A., Bhopal, R., & SHELS researchers. (2016). Ethnic variations in asthma hospital admission, readmission and death: A retrospective, national cohort study of 4.62 million people in Scotland. *BMC Medicine, 14*, 3.

Sundmacher, L., Fischbach, D., Schuettig, W., Naumann, C., Augustin, U., & Faisst, C. (2015). Which hospitalisations are ambulatory care-sensitive, to what degree, and how could the rates be reduced? Results of a group consensus study in Germany. *Health Policy, 119*, 1415–1423. https://doi.org/10.1016/j.healthpol.2015.08.007.

United Nations, Department of Economic and Social Affairs, Population Division. International Migration Report 2015 (ST/ESA/SER.A/384). (2015).

United Nations. World Economic Situation and Prospects. (2016). http://www.un.org/en/development/desa/policy/wesp/wesp_current/2016wesp_full_en.pdf. Accessed 3 July 2017.

Urquia, M. L., Glazier, R. H., Blondel, B., Zeitlin, J., Gissler, M., Macfarlane, A., et al. (2010). International migration and adverse birth outcomes: Role of ethnicity, region of origin and destination. *Journal of Epidemiology and Community Health, 64*, 243–251. https://doi.org/10.1136/jech.2008.083535.

van Loenen, T., Faber, M. J., Westert, G. P., & Van den Berg, M. J. (2016). The impact of primary care organization on avoidable hospital admissions for diabetes in 23 countries. *Scandinavian Journal of Primary Health Care, 34*, 5–12. https://doi.org/10.3109/02813432.2015.1132883.

van Loenen, T., van den Berg, M. J., Westert, G. P., & Faber, M. J. (2014). Organizational aspects of primary care related to hospitalization: A systematic review. *Family Practice, 31*, 502–516. https://doi.org/10.1093/fampra/cmu053.

Wagstaff, A. (2009). Social health insurance vs. tax-financed health systems – evidence from the OECD. Policy Research working paper; no. WPS 4821. Washington, DC: World Bank Group.

Walker, R. L., Ghali, W. A., Chen, G., Khalsa, T. K., Mangat, B. K., Campbell, N. R. C., et al. (2017). ACSC indicator: Testing reliability for hypertension. *BMC Medical Informatics and Decision Making, 17*, 90. https://doi.org/10.1186/s12911-017-0487-4.

Weeks, W. B., Ventelou, B., & Paraponaris, A. (2016). Rates of admission for ambulatory care sensitive conditions in France in 2009–2010: Trends, geographic variation, costs, and an international comparison. *The European Journal of Health Economics, 17*, 453–470. https://doi.org/10.1007/s10198-015-0692-y.

WHO Europe. (2017). Migration and health: key issues. http://www.euro.who.int/en/health-topics/health-determinants/migration-and-health/migrant-health-in-the-european-region/migration-and-health-key-issues#292115. Accessed 5 July 2017.

Wild, S., Roglic, G., Green, A., Sicree, R., & King, H. (2004). Global prevalence of diabetes: Estimates for the year 2000 and projections for 2030. *Diabetes Care, 27*, 1047–1053.

William, G., & Noori, T. (2014). Infectious disease burden in migrant populations in the EU and EEA. In: Migrants and health. *European Journal of Public Health, 20*, 3–6.

Wright, B., Potter, A. J., & Trivedi, A. N. (2017). Use of federally qualified health centers and potentially preventable hospital utilization among older Medicare-Medicaid enrollees. *The Journal of Ambulatory Care Management, 40*, 139–149. https://doi.org/10.1097/JAC.0000000000000158.

Yam, C. H., Wong, E. L., Chan, F. W., Wong, F. Y., Leung, M. C., & Yeoh, E. K. (2010 Oct). Measuring and preventing potentially avoidable hospital readmissions: A review of the literature. *Hong Kong Medical Journal, 16*(5), 383–389.

Chapter 8
Adaptation of Primary Health Care for Migrants: Recommendations and Best Practices

Marie Dauvrin and Bernadett Varga

8.1 Introduction

Worldwide, there is a consensus about the need for adapting primary health care for migrants but the way to achieve this aim may be hazardous for those willing to enter the field without any safety net (WHO Regional Office for Europe 2010). There are many interventions, recommendations and guidelines to reduce disparities in access and in outcomes for migrants but not all these interventions are evidence-based, nor are they what one may call a best practice. And this takes place in a particularly challenging context as migrants constitute a heterogeneous group of individuals, with various needs and profiles, evolving over time.

Moreover, interventions could not be isolated from their sociocultural and political context, the resources available, and the attitudes and behaviors of both migrants and professionals. Adapting health care does not necessarily mean that there is a need for creating new services or ensuring that migrants are able to use the services as everybody else: adapting the existing offer may be sufficient but one may thus be particularly careful when adapting primary health care services to migrants (WHO Regional Office for Europe 2010).

M. Dauvrin (✉)
Institute of Health and Society, Université catholique de Louvain, Brussels, Belgium

Parnasse-ISEI, Haute Ecole Léonard de Vinci, Brussels, Belgium
e-mail: marie.dauvrin@uclouvain.be

B. Varga
Institute of Health and Society, Université catholique de Louvain, Brussels, Belgium
e-mail: marie.dauvrin@uclouvain.be

© The Author(s), under exclusive licence to Springer International Publishing AG,
part of Springer Nature 2018
A. Rosano (ed.), *Access to Primary Care and Preventative Health Services of Migrants*,
SpringerBriefs in Public Health, https://doi.org/10.1007/978-3-319-73630-3_8

Best practice and cultural competence

A best practice in adapting primary health care for migrants should be a culturally-competent practice. There are numerous definitions and models of cultural competence but the most widely acknowledged is the definition proposed by Cross and colleagues: *"a set of congruent behaviors, attitudes, and policies that come together in a system, agency, or among professionals and enable that system, agency or those professionals to work effectively in cross-cultural situations. The word "culture" is used because it implies the integrated pattern of human behavior that include thoughts, communications, actions, customs, beliefs, values, and institutions of a racial, ethnic, religious, or social group. The word competence is used because it implies having the capacity to function effectively. A culturally competent system of care incorporates – at all levels – the importance of culture, the assessment of cross-cultural relations, vigilance towards the dynamics that result from cultural differences, the expansion of cultural knowledge, and the adaptation of services to meet culturally-unique needs"* (Retrieved from Cross et al. 1989, p. 13).

8.1.1 What Constitutes a Best Practice in Primary Health Care?

There is no single answer to this crucial question. However, from an equity lens, a best practice should be an intervention – in the broader sense – aiming a gradually reducing all systematic differences in health between migrants and the rest of the population (Adapted from Whitehead and Dahlgren 2007). It could take the form of a direct service provision to a patient but also be a health policy or a program for health care professionals. As stated by Whitehead & Dahlgren, achieving equity in health lies on *levelling up* the population to the same health outcomes than the most privileged (Whitehead and Dahlgren 2007).

Adapting primary care, and thus achieving equity, will then require an intersectional and multisectoral approach to cope with the diversity of the migrants and to level them up (WHO Regional Office for Europe 2010). Hankivsky postulates that *"intersectionality promotes an understanding of human beings as shaped by the interaction of different social locations (e.g., 'race'/ethnicity, Indigeneity, gender, class, sexuality, geography, age, disability/ability, migration status, religion). These interactions occur within a context of connected systems and structures of power (e.g., laws, policies, state governments and other political and economic unions, religious institutions, media). Through such processes, interdependent forms of privilege and oppression shaped by colonialism, imperialism, racism, homophobia, ableism and patriarchy are created."*(Hankivsky 2014; Hankivsky et al. 2014) This requires then from those adapting services not only to focus on the migrant aspect but on other social determinants and characteristics of the targeted group. Oliver et al. (2008) proposed the typology PROGRESS+ to identify the multiple characteristics of a patient group (Oliver et al. 2008).

PROGRESS Plus

The PROGRESS Plus framework is a mnemonic tool used to categorize populations. It consists of:

- **P** Place of residence: Rural/urban, country/state, area deprivation, housing characteristics
- **Religion** Religious background
- **Occupation** Professional, skilled, unskilled, unemployed etc.
- **Gender** Male or female
- **Race/Ethnicity** Ethnic background
- **Education** Years in and/or level of education attained, school type
- **Social capital** Neighborhood/community/family support
- **Socio-economic status** (SES) Income-related measure e.g. means-tested benefits/welfare, affluence measures etc.
- **Plus**

  - **Age**
  - **Disability** Existence of physical or emotional/mental disability
  - **Sexual orientation** Heterosexual, gay, lesbian, bisexual, transgender

  Content of the categories could be determined by the ones using it. For example, ethnicity could be defined by variables such as country of birth, migration status, spoken languages, preferred language, citizenship, length of stay or level of acculturation (Aspinall 2007).

One may thus argue that there is no venue to develop group interventions and that each intervention should be unique and individualized. However, this is neither desirable nor sustainable for any health care system. A best practice will be thus a practice supporting both horizontal and vertical equity. Horizontal equity means ensuring that all migrants have the same access to primary care service while the vertical equity considers the specific needs of migrants and thus adapts the health care system accordingly. Vertical equity is sometimes used as a synonym for what scholars also call "*responsiveness*", defined by Bischoff as "*responsiveness to the socio-cultural background of migrant and minority patients, focusing on hospitals' positive responses to their needs. Responsiveness also includes the adequacy of health care facilities in meeting the needs of migrant and minority patients, including both structural aspects of hospitals and training for health professionals*" (Bischoff 2003).

8.1.2 Users' Involvement: The Key to Success

How should one then know which patient characteristic needs to be the center of attention? By involving the patients and the community in the decision-making and the process of adaption of services. This is one of the recommendations made by the WHO while addressing migrant health (WHO Regional Office for Europe 2010).

At the start of every project, four attention points need to be considered: (1) users may be tired of being consulted; (2) "professional" patients – monopolizing the room at the detriment of other patients less often involved; (3) lack of acknowledgement of the patients – supporting the need for finding efficient incentives; (4) fear – not only among patients but also among health care professionals that may feel insecure if they anticipated that their practices may be questioned (Brady et al. 2007) .

Besides, the project initiators may need to perform their self-assessment regarding the users' involvement before the start. This evaluation may encompass dimensions such as leadership and involvement, practices and procedures, approach to users, training and resources, quality and evaluation practices…. Checklists such as the Scottish Checking for Change or the Migrant-Friendly Hospitals may be of interest.

A wide range of participative methods help the professionals to involve the patients (and their relatives) in the adaptation of services, the main difficulty being choosing the most adapted one. Five criteria guide the decision (King Baudouin Fundation 2006):

1. Objectives – why do you need a participative approach? Some distinguish the objectives between the motivation (democratization versus advices) and the outcome (organizing diversity versus looking for a consensus)
2. Topic – what is the nature and the amplitude of the issue concerned?
3. Users – who is concerned with the issue, interested in or likely to contribute to the solutions?
4. Duration – what time period is available for setting up the process?
5. Resources – what are the available resources (budget, staff, equipment…)?

8.2 Where Do You Find Examples of Recommendations and Best Practices?

The distinction we made between the different levels of the health care system is a theoretical distinction: one may not hope to achieve best practices in primary care by focusing solely on one level of the health care system. Cultural competence results from the interactions between the different levels and should be considered as a process of both personal and organizational change.

8.2.1 Adaptations at Individual Level

8.2.1.1 Communication

Barriers due to linguistic and language differences are often considered by the health care professionals as the most frequent but also the most difficult challenge to overcome (Dauvrin and Lorant 2014; Bischoff 2012). In presence of linguistic barriers, there is an increased risk of non-adherence to treatment or recommendations, diagnosis delays or errors, misuse of services, inappropriate treatments, unnecessary tests, delayed care, poor satisfaction of both patients and health care professionals to cite a few (Bischoff 2003; Bischoff and Hudelson 2010a; Scheppers et al. 2006). Consequently, improving communication is often perceived as a priority area for adapting services and has been widely recommended by experts (Deville et al. 2011; Pottie et al. 2014; Meeuwesen et al. 2012).

Moreover, health care professionals declare being responsible for adapting communication rather than putting this responsibility on the migrants –by involving interpreters, or by providing written information in an adapted language (Hudelson et al. 2010; Dauvrin and Lorant 2014). Those willing to adapt their services may begin by solving the language issues. Once an efficient communication channel has been established, the health care professional and the patient may engage in a positive relationship. Working with an interpreter therefore requires following some guidelines to ensure an effective communication.

> **Ten tips for working with an interpreter**
> Hieroglifs Translations made a funny and accessible video summarizing the 10 tips to work with an interpreter that may be used as didactic material. The video link is available at the following URL: https://www.youtube.com/watch?v=ABn0sE1aiGo

Having an interpreter is not always feasible or accessible for primary care practices, unless the service is confronted with the same migrant group for years. However, in practice, as migration is a dynamic process, it is unrealistic to have interpreters for all languages. Recently, interpreting services by videoconference have shown promising results as it broadens the spectrum of available languages, necessitates only a connected device (but preferably a computer with a large size screen), and is easy to organize. Videoconference interpreting therefore requires the same preparation as face-to-face interpreting. When adequately deployed, (video) interpreting increases access to health care, patient and professional satisfaction and reduces costs for the institution (Bischoff and Hudelson 2010a, b).

If interpreting addresses language barriers, it may not be sufficient when cultural issues are at play (Bischoff and Hudelson 2010b). A best practice is thus to involve intercultural mediators that will take care of both language and cultural issues (Verrept 2012; Baraldi and Gavioli 2012). Besides interpreting, intercultural mediators also act as cultural bridges between the patients (and their relatives) and the health care professionals by eliciting health beliefs and values, cultural and/or religious aspects as well as other elements that may influence the relationship. They also participate in patient education, patient advocacy, counselling but also in the training activities for health care professionals. Belgium, Italy, the United States or Canada have been using (inter)cultural mediators for years and it shows positive outcomes on patient and professional satisfaction (Nierkens et al. 2002; Verrept 2012; Baraldi and Gavioli 2012). Moreover, intercultural mediators are often members of the migrant communities and may support the social integration and the valorization of their competences in the wider society.

Improving communication may also be supported by additional tools: using pictograms, displaying information posters in various languages, having flyers in the most spoken languages. In that sense, schools, community centers, NGO and other non-profit organizations are partners that may help the primary care facility to create a friendly space. When holding a consultation with an interpreter / mediator, a sign on the door may prevent from being interrupted.

Communication can also be improved by providing health care professional with the ability to communicate directly with the patients in their own languages. This may be achieved by promoting access to health care professions among migrants, encouraging diplomas equivalencies through agreements among countries, migrant-oriented recruitment policies in health care services – this kind of policy has therefore to be strictly regulated to avoid a negative impact on the health system of the country of origin of the migrants-, (financial) incentives for bilingual workers, or institutional database of language spoken by health care professionals.

Although this last initiative is quite low-cost and easy to develop, it needs to be reserved for emergency situations to prevent inadequate situations like using non-qualified personal (e.g. cleaning staff is not adequate for interpreting) or monopolizing a health care professional for interpreting and not caring. As an illustration, a negative situation was experienced by a hospital nurse being the only one speaking Aramean in her institution: she became monopolized by interpreting instead of performing her caring duties. This led to tensions and finally the nurse refused to interpret (Dauvrin 2013).

Communication improvement on the patient side could be achieved through integration classes or (compulsory) language classes. These initiatives are therefore feasible for newcomers and are rather difficult to implement with migrants living in the country for years. Partnership between associations promoting (health) literacy and health care services must be considered.

8.2.1.2   Culturally Sensitive Health Promotion

Health promotion activities are at heart of the primary care services and are of importance with migrant populations. Culturally sensitive health promotion requires adaptations in the conception, the planning, the promotion, the recruitment of participants, the implementation, the retention and the evaluation process. Liu et al. underwent a major evidence synthesis in 2012 aiming at identifying how to adapt health promotion interventions to the needs of ethnic minority groups and listed all the adaptations likely to suit the needs of migrant populations (Liu et al. 2012). Culturally sensitive health promotion is highly context-dependent but five common principles of adaptation are at stake, whatever the topic or the target group involved: *"(1) Drawing on community resources for promotion and increasing accessibility; (2) Identifying barriers to access and participation; (3) Developing language – and format -appropriate strategies; (4) Utilizing cultural and/or religious values for strategies that promote change; (5) Accommodating for different levels of cultural identification"* (Liu et al. 2012, p. 13).

Culturally sensitive health promotion therefore requires a cautious approach if the final objective is to improve equity for all. A common pitfall is that the intervention reduces the disparities inside the migrant group and not among migrants and the rest of the population. To ensure the equity of the interventions, Tugwell et al. (2010) proposed an equity-oriented analytical framework organized around seven dimensions: (1) developing an intervention model; (2) defining disadvantage; (3) deciding on appropriate study design(s); (4) identifying outcomes of interest; (5) process evaluation and understanding context; (6) analyzing and presenting data, and (7) judging the applicability of results (Tugwell et al. 2010).

8.2.1.3 Health Literacy

Improving health literacy should be a transversal objective of improving communication and providing culturally sensitive health promotion as health literacy is of crucial importance for the most vulnerable ones such as migrants. Indeed, individuals with an appropriate level of health literacy will be more likely to, i.e., participate in preventive and screening activities, adopt healthy behaviors, be compliant, prevent chronic diseases or take decisions for their health. Figure 8.1 illustrates the dimensions of health literacy (Van Den Broucke and Renwart 2014).

Interventions in health literacy lay on five characteristics: (1) a global and positive vision of health, (2) a collective approach, (3) a proximity approach, (4) a lifelong approach and (5) actions targeting the individual and its environment (Cultures&Santé 2016). They concern different issues such as health determinants, health systems and social welfare systems, risk factors and protective factors related to a disease or an accident and diseases, health and healthcare. The content will be determined in accordance with the migrant needs. For example, newcomers may

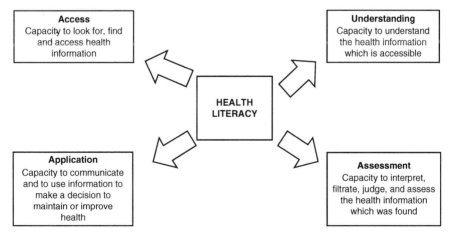

Fig. 8.1 Dimensions of health literacy (Adapted and translated from Van Den Broucke and Renwart (2014))

benefit from interventions presenting the health and social welfare systems while a second-generation migrant may be more interested in health determinants. The objective of the intervention, i.e. smoking cessation versus adopting a healthy diet, also influences the approach and the materials used (Taggart et al. 2012). Assessing health literacy needs is helped by tools such as the Health Literacy Skills Instrument, the Short Test of Functional Health Literacy in Adults, or instruments tailored to a specific health condition (Al Sayah et al. 2013; Hersh et al. 2015; Bann et al. 2012). Fernandez-Gutierrez and colleagues found therefore few interventions tailored to migrant populations (Fernandez-Gutierrez et al. 2017). Recommendations for primary care practices exist about verbal communication, numeracy and written materials but will need adaptations to the linguistic barriers (Hersh et al. 2015).

Collective and individual interactions, information supports, audiovisual campaigns, numeric supports are among the numerous channels that may be used to support health literacy interventions but, again, the final intervention will be context-dependent (Taggart et al. 2012; Hersh et al. 2015). Taggart and colleagues found, i.e., that the place of delivery plays a role in the effectiveness: smoking cessation is more effective in a primary care service while changing nutrition or physical activity is better supported in community settings (Taggart et al. 2012). They also found that the intensity of the intervention did not impact its effectiveness (Taggart et al. 2012). Again, those willing to develop such interventions will have to carefully assess the needs and the resources available. Engaging with associations promoting literacy and numeracy may be a key asset for primary care services willing to develop health literacy activities with their patients. Moreover, Adsul and colleagues recommended having a dedicated professional in charge of health literacy activities to support organizational changes (Adsul et al. 2017).

8.2.2 Adaptations at Organizational Level

8.2.2.1 Training of Health Care Professionals

Improving the competencies of health care professionals through training has been widely recommended over the years and, consequently, a large spectrum of studies try to cover this field. Content of the training programs may include patient-centered care, self-knowledge and personal development, interpersonal communication and soft skills, immersion in "cultural" environments or specific knowledge on migrants. This last point has been the most controversial as it may increase stereotypes and prejudices against migrants (Seeleman et al. 2009; Chiarenza 2012). The temptation was great to have "recipes" indicating how to behave with a well-defined migrant group. Examples of such recipes were "how to greet a Muslim", "how to handle sadness with a Chinese" or "how to talk with a Catholic". However, this "cookbook" approach does not consider that heterogeneity is equally important inside a migrant "group" as between migrant groups. Socioeconomic factors also contribute to the diversity and the vulnerability of migrants, leading to a unique and personal health experience.

The most striking examples are related to the impact of religious beliefs or alimentary customs: not all Africans eat *foufou*, not all Muslims practice Ramadan. Consequently, the most efficient training programs are those promoting interdisciplinary and intersectoral work, patient-centered care and other soft-skills oriented programs. These will not only support effective care with migrants but also with other (vulnerable) patients, improving equity for all. The MEM-TP project, funded by the European Commission, realized a review of existing training materials and suggested additional training packages for health professionals (Chiarenza et al. 2015).

Recommendations for developing training package for health care professionals (adapted from (Chiarenza et al. 2015))

Individual development

- Promote the construction of argumentative knowledge and collaborative learning
- Promote training that addresses a multi-professional and multi-disciplinary audience
- Develop a clear rationale and a consistent pedagogical approach for the training program
- Embed a focus on outcomes in training design, delivery and evaluation methods

Organizational development

- Develop a diversity responsiveness management framework
- Develop a diversity responsiveness assessment framework
- Ensure training is linked to organizational policy and support mechanisms
- Allocate appropriate resource funding to the training

Community development

- Promote cooperation and integration between health services and relevant stakeholders
- Involve service users and stakeholders in training planning, development and evaluation

Policy development

- Embed training in policy and legislative requirements
- Promote the implementation of a whole-organization and health-system approach
- Promote the engagement of university, government agencies and international organizations
- Promote the systematic training of health care professionals in schools and having curricula systematically addressing these issues

Similarly, the format of these trainings encompasses a wide range of possibilities. Some countries have a long tradition of including cultural competence in the initial training of all health professionals while, in other countries, cultural competence is part of the lifelong education, the former being the exception. As evidenced by the 2015 MIPEX inventory, health care staff benefit from a nationally organized training regarding migrants' health in only four countries: United Kingdom, Norway, New-Zealand and Switzerland (Huddleston et al. 2015).

But, independently of the content and the format, the key to sustainable cultural competence is to have a strong institutional commitment and a positive leadership regarding migrants. The most culturally competent nurse performing in an environment where there is no room for cultural competence is useless. Similarly, a health care professional whose competences and skills are acknowledged by the institution is most likely to use them when caring for a migrant patient and, by the role-modeling and leadership, may influence his/her colleagues (Dauvrin and Lorant 2017, 2015). The effects of (culturally competent) training decrease over time when not deployed in a supportive work environment. To be effective, the skills and competences acquired through training need to be valued and valorized (Barnes et al. 2013). Social learning is equally important in the development of cultural competence of health care professionals, particularly as these are mostly non-technical skills (Curry et al. 2011). Leaders – both formal or informal- and cultural competence champions play a major role in spreading cultural competences, more than peers (Dauvrin and Lorant 2017, 2015).

8.2.2.2 Interdisciplinary and Intersectoral Work

To improve equity of services for migrants, the WHO recommended to better involve the NGOs, experts and community workers. As stated earlier, the adaptation of primary care services requires an interdisciplinary and intersectoral approach. Pottie et al. (2014) defined intersectoral approach as *"a strategy consisting of coordinated actions between the health sector and health services, as well as other stakeholders and sectors of society (education, industry, sanitation, environment, etc.), working together to achieve specific health goals for the population"* (Pottie et al. 2014, page e38). As an example, in Oslo, Jenum et al. successfully implemented an intersectoral program promoting physical activity among a multiethnic population (Jenum et al. 2006).

However, as goals, objectives and methods are likely to differ between the different actors, there is a need for formalization, through formalization tools and regular information exchange (D'Amour et al. 2008). Agreements between services may help to clarify the missions and to ensure a shared vision. As an illustration, in Brussels, a primary care service (private service) established a partnership with a community center (public service). The physiotherapist of the primary care service organizes relaxation and yoga classes in a room loaned by the community center. The social worker of the community center holds permanence at the primary care

Table 8.1 A good interdisciplinary team (Nancarrow et al. 2013)

Themes	Description
1. Leadership and management	Having a clear leader of the team, with clear direction and management; democratic; shared power; support/supervision; personal development aligned with line management; leader who acts and listens
2. Communication	Individuals with communication skills; ensuring that there are appropriate systems to promote communication with the team
3. Personal rewards, training and development	Learning, training and development; training and career development opportunities; incorporate individual rewards and opportunity, morale and motivation
4. Appropriate resources and procedures	Structures (for example, team meetings, organizational factors, team members working from the same location). Ensuring that appropriate procedures are in place to uphold the vision of the service (for example, communication systems, appropriate referral criteria and so on).
5. Appropriate skill mix	Sufficient/appropriate skills, competencies, practitioner mix, balance of personalities; ability to make the most of other team members' backgrounds; having a full complement of staff; timely replacement/ cover for empty or absent posts.
6. Climate	Team culture of trust, valuing contributions, nurturing consensus; need to create an interprofessional atmosphere
7. Individual characteristics	Knowledge, experience, initiatives, knowing strengths and weaknesses, listening skills, reflexive practice; desire to work on the same goals
8. Clarity of vision	Having a clear set of values that drive the direction of the service and the care provided. Portraying a uniform and consistent external image.
9. Quality of outcomes of care	Patient-centered focus, outcomes and satisfaction, encouraging feedback, capturing and recording evidence of effectiveness of care, and using that as part of a feedback cycle to improve care
10. Respecting and understanding roles	Sharing power, joint working, autonomy

service. Once a year, a general assembly gathers the personal of the community center and the primary care service. To ensure the collaboration, an agreement, including aspects related to patient confidentiality, was written and accepted by all members (Dauvrin 2013).

If interdisciplinary is considered as an evidence-based practice in adapting health care for migrants, professionals are not (always) trained about how to put into practice (Beach et al. 2005). Based on a systematic review and interviews with professionals, Nancarrow et al. (2013) identified the ten characteristics of what constitutes a good interdisciplinary team (Nancarrow et al. 2013) (Table 8.1).

8.3 Adaptations at Structural Level

Adaptations at the structural level relate to the political and institutional context: this requires a clear acknowledgement that diversity is part of the national identity and that attention should be devoted to migrants. Despite recommendations from the United Nations, the WHO, the Council of Europe or the European Union, inclusion of migrants still remains heterogeneously implemented (Council of Europe 2006; WHO Regional Office for Europe 2010; WHO 2008).

Recommendations for responsive primary health care services
- Checking for Change, NHS Scotland
- Culturally and Linguistically Appropriate Services (CLAS) standards, Office of Minority health, United States
- Equity standards, Health Promoting Hospitals; Task Force on Migrant-Friendly and Culturally Competent Health care, Europe
- Migrant Friendly Hospitals, Europe
- Joint Commission Roadmap, The Joint Commission, United States
- Cultural Responsiveness Framework, Victorian Government, Australia
- Council of Europe Recommendations, Committee of Ministers, Council of Europe
- Equality Delivery System, The Equality and Diversity Council, United Kingdom
- ETHEALTH, Ministry of Public Health, Belgium

This heterogeneity is therefore only at the implementation level (McCalman et al. 2017). By comparing six standards for responsive health services, Seeleman et al. (2015) showed that there is a consensus about what should be a responsive health service: *"organizational commitment, collecting and analyzing data to provide empirical evidence on inequalities and needs, development of a competent and diverse workforce, ensuring access for all users, ensuring responsiveness in care provision, fostering patient and community participation, and actively promoting the ideal of responsiveness* (Seeleman et al. 2015).

8.4   Conclusion

This chapter aimed at providing guidance to those interested in adapting their primary care services to the needs of their migrant patients. There is no magical formula, each intervention will have to be tailored to the context, the migrants, the professionals and the resources available. Adapting primary care services will take time and must be considered as an iterative process to cope with the dynamic aspect of migration: nothing should be definitive and the health care system should always be responsive to achieve equity for all.

References

Adsul, P., Wray, R., Gautam, K., Jupka, K., Weaver, N., & Wilson, K. (2017). Becoming a health literate organization: Formative research results from healthcare organizations providing care for undeserved communities. *Health Services Management Research*: 951484817727130. doi:https://doi.org/10.1177/0951484817727130.

Al Sayah, F., Williams, B., & Johnson, J. A. (2013). Measuring health literacy in individuals with diabetes: A systematic review and evaluation of available measures. *Health Education & Behavior: The Official Publication of the Society for Public Health Education, 40*(1), 42–55. https://doi.org/10.1177/1090198111436341

Aspinall, P. J. (2007). Approaches to developing an improved cross-national understanding of concepts and terms relating to ethnicity and race. *International Sociology, 22*(1), 41–70. https://doi.org/10.1177/0268580907070124

Bann, C. M., McCormack, L. A., Berkman, N. D., & Squiers, L. B. (2012). The health literacy skills instrument: A 10-item short form. *Journal of Health Communication, 17*(Suppl 3), 191–202. https://doi.org/10.1080/10810730.2012.718042

Baraldi, C., & Gavioli, L. (2012). Assessing linguistic and cultural mediation in healthcare services. In D. Ingleby, A. Chiarenza, W. Deville, & I. Kotsioni (Eds.), *Inequalities in health care for migrants and ethnic minorities* (Vol. 2, pp. 144–157). Antwerpen: Garant.

Barnes, E., Bullock, A. D., Bailey, S. E., Cowpe, J. G., & Karaharju-Suvanto, T. (2013). A review of continuing professional development for dentists in Europe(*). *European Journal of Dental Education: Official Journal of the Association for Dental Education in Europe, 17*(Suppl 1), 5–17. https://doi.org/10.1111/eje.12045

Beach, M. C., Price, E. G., Gary, T. L., Robinson, K. A., Gozu, A., Palacio, A., Smarth, C., Jenckes, M. W., Feuerstein, C., Bass, E. B., Powe, N. R., & Cooper, L. A. (2005). Cultural competence: A systematic review of health care provider educational interventions. *Medical Care, 43*(4), 356–373.

Bischoff, A. (2003). *Caring for migrant and minority patients in European hospitals. A review of effective interventions*. Neuchâtel and Basel: Swiss Forum for Migration and Populations Studies.

Bischoff, A. (2012). Do language barriers increase inequalities? Do interprets decrease inequalities? In D. Ingleby, A. Chiarenza, W. Deville, & I. Kotsioni (Eds.), *Inequalities in health care for migrants and ethnic minorities* (Vol. 2, pp. 128–143). Antwerpen: Garant.

Bischoff, A., & Hudelson, P. (2010a). Access to healthcare interpreter services: Where are we and where do we need to go? *International Journal of Environmental Research and Public Health, 7*(7), 2838–2844. https://doi.org/10.3390/ijerph7072838

Bischoff, A., & Hudelson, P. (2010b). Communicating with foreign language-speaking patients: Is access to professional interpreters enough? *Journal of Travel Medicine, 17*(1), 15–20. https://doi.org/10.1111/j.1708-8305.2009.00314.x

Brady, B., Lescrauwaet, D., Latour, N., Carlson, J., & Kneip, R. (2007). Participation toolkit. Redistributing the power! European Federation of National Organisations working with the homeless, Brussels.

Chiarenza, A. (2012). Development in the concept of "cultural competence". In D. Ingleby, A. Chiarenza, W. Devillé, & I. Kotsioni (Eds.), *Inequalities in health care for migrants and ethnic minorities* (Vol. 2, pp. 66–81). Antwerpen: Garant.

Chiarenza, A., Horvat, L., Ciannameo, A., Vaccaro, G., Lanting, K., Bodewes, A., & Suurmond, J. (2015). Training materials development: Review of existing training materials. Work package 2. Training package for health professionals to improve access and quality of health services for migrants and ethnic minorities, including the Roma MEM-TP. Azienda Unita Sanitaria Locale di Reggio Emilia, Academic Medical Centre – University of Amsterdam, Brussels.

Council of Europe. (2006). *Recommendation Rec(2006)18 of the Committee of Ministers to member states on health services in a multicultural society vol Rec(2006)18*. Strasbourg: Council of Europe.

Cross, T., Bazron, B., Dennis, K., & Isaacs, M. R. (1989). Towards a culturally competent system of care. CASSP (Ed.). Georgetown: Georgetown University Child Development Center.

Cultures&Santé. (2016). *La littératie en santé: D'un concept à la pratique [Health literacy: from concept to practice]*. Brussels: Cultures&Santé.

Curry, S. E., Cortland, C. I., & Graham, M. J. (2011). Role-modelling in the operating room: Medical student observations of exemplary behaviour. *Medical Education, 45*(9), 946–957. https://doi.org/10.1111/j.1365-2923.2011.04014.x

D'Amour, D., Goulet, L., Labadie, J. F., Martin-Rodriguez, L. S., & Pineault, R. (2008). A model and typology of collaboration between professionals in healthcare organizations. *BMC Health Services Research, 8*, 188. https://doi.org/10.1186/1472-6963-8-188

Dauvrin, M. (2013). *Cultural competence in health care: Challenging inequalities, involving institutions*. Brussels: Université catholique de Louvain.

Dauvrin, M., & Lorant, V. (2014). Adaptation of health care for migrants: Whose responsibility? *BMC Health Services Research, 14*, 294. https://doi.org/10.1186/1472-6963-14-294

Dauvrin, M., & Lorant, V. (2015). Leadership and cultural competence of healthcare professionals: A social network analysis. *Nursing Research, 64*(3), 200–210. https://doi.org/10.1097/NNR.0000000000000092

Dauvrin, M., & Lorant, V. (2017). Cultural competence and social relationships: A social network analysis. *International Nursing Review, 64*(2), 195–204. https://doi.org/10.1111/inr.12327

Deville, W., Greacen, T., Bogic, M., Dauvrin, M., Dias, S., Gaddini, A., Jensen, N. K., Karamanidou, C., Kluge, U., Mertaniemi, R., Riera, R. P., Sarvary, A., Soares, J. J., Stankunas, M., Strassmayr, C., Welbel, M., & Priebe, S. (2011). Health care for immigrants in Europe: Is there still consensus among country experts about principles of good practice? A Delphi study. *BMC Public Health, 11*, 699. https://doi.org/10.1186/1471-2458-11-699

Fernandez-Gutierrez, M., Bas-Sarmiento, P., Albar-Marin, M. J., Paloma-Castro, O., & Romero-Sanchez, J. M. (2017) Health literacy interventions for immigrant populations: A systematic review. *International Nursing Review*. Epub ahead of print. doi:https://doi.org/10.1111/inr.12373.

Hankivsky, O. (2014). *Intersectionality 101*. Vancouver: The Institute for Intersectionality Research & Policy, SFU.

Hankivsky, O., Grace, D., Hunting, G., Giesbrecht, M., Fridkin, A., Rudrum, S., Ferlatte, O., & Clark, N. (2014). An intersectionality-based policy analysis framework: Critical reflections on a methodology for advancing equity. *International Journal for Equity in Health, 13*, 119. https://doi.org/10.1186/s12939-014-0119-x

Hersh, L., Salzman, B., & Snyderman, D. (2015). Health literacy in primary care practice. *American Family Physician, 92*(2), 118–124.

Huddleston, T., Bilgili, Ö., Joki, A.-L., & Vankova, Z. (2015). *Migrant integration policy index 2015*. Barcelona/Brussels: CIDOB and MPG.

Hudelson, P., Perron, N. J., & Perneger, T. V. (2010). Measuring physicians' and medical students' attitudes toward caring for immigrant patients. *Evaluation & the Health Professions, 33*(4), 452–472. https://doi.org/10.1177/0163278710370157

Jenum, A. K., Anderssen, S. A., Birkeland, K. I., Holme, I., Graff-Iversen, S., Lorentzen, C., Ommundsen, Y., Raastad, T., Odegaard, A. K., & Bahr, R. (2006). Promoting physical activity in a low-income multiethnic district: Effects of a community intervention study to reduce risk factors for type 2 diabetes and cardiovascular disease: A community intervention reducing inactivity. *Diabetes Care, 29*(7), 1605–1612. https://doi.org/10.2337/dc05-1587

King Baudouin Foundation. (2006). *Participatory methods toolkit. A practitioner's manual*. Brussels: King Baudouin Foundation.

Liu, J., Davidson, E., Bhopal, R., White, M., Johnson, M., Netto, G., Deverill, M., & Sheikh, A. (2012). Adapting health promotion interventions to meet the needs of ethnic minority groups: Mixed-methods evidence synthesis. *Health Technology Assessment, 16*(44), 1–469. https://doi.org/10.3310/hta16440

McCalman, J., Jongen, C., & Bainbridge, R. (2017). Organisational systems' approaches to improving cultural competence in healthcare: A systematic scoping review of the literature. *International Journal for Equity in Health, 16*(1), 78. https://doi.org/10.1186/s12939-017-0571-5

Meeuwesen, L., Ekpenying, A., Cesaroni, F., Eversley, J., & Ross, J. (2012). Interpreting in health and social care : Policies and interventions in five European countries. In D. Ingleby, A. Chiarenza, W. Deville, & I. Kotsioni (Eds.), *Inequalities in health care for migrants and ethnic minorities* (Vol. 2, pp. 158–172). Antwerpen: Garant.

Nancarrow, S. A., Booth, A., Ariss, S., Smith, T., Enderby, P., & Roots, A. (2013). Ten principles of good interdisciplinary team work. *Human Resources for Health, 11*, 19. https://doi.org/10.1186/1478-4491-11-19

Nierkens, V., Krumeich, A., de Ridder, R., & van Dongen, M. (2002). The future of intercultural mediation in Belgium. *Patient Education and Counseling, 46*(4), 253–259.

Oliver, S., Kavanagh, J., Caird, J., Lorenc, T., Oliver, K., Harden, A., Thomas, J., Greaves, A., & Oakley, A. (2008). *Health promotion, inequalities and young people's health. A systematic review of research.* Vol EPPI-Centre report no. 1611. London: EPPI-Centre, Social Science Research Unit, Institute of Education, University of London.

Pottie, K., Batista, R., Mayhew, M., Mota, L., & Grant, K. (2014). Improving delivery of primary care for vulnerable migrants: Delphi consensus to prioritize innovative practice strategies. *Canadian Family Physician Medecin De Famille Canadien, 60*(1), e32–e40.

Scheppers, E., van Dongen, E., Dekker, J., Geertzen, J., & Dekker, J. (2006). Potential barriers to the use of health services among ethnic minorities: A review. *Family Practice, 23*(3), 325–348. https://doi.org/10.1093/fampra/cmi113

Seeleman, C., Suurmond, J., & Stronks, K. (2009). Cultural competence: A conceptual framework for teaching and learning. *Medical Education, 43*(3), 229–237. https://doi.org/10.1111/j.1365-2923.2008.03269.x

Seeleman, C., Essink-Bot, M.-L., Stronks, K., & Ingleby, D. (2015). How should health service organizations respond to diversity? A content analysis of six approaches. *BMC Health Services Research, 15*, 510. https://doi.org/10.1186/s12913-015-1159-7

Taggart, J., Williams, A., Dennis, S., Newall, A., Shortus, T., Zwar, N., Denney-Wilson, E., & Harris, M. F. (2012). A systematic review of interventions in primary care to improve health literacy for chronic disease behavioral risk factors. *BMC Family Practice, 13*, 49. https://doi.org/10.1186/1471-2296-13-49

Tugwell, P., Petticrew, M., Kristjansson, E., Welch, V., Ueffing, E., Waters, E., Bonnefoy, J., Morgan, A., Doohan, E., & Kelly, M. P. (2010). Assessing equity in systematic reviews: Realising the recommendations of the commission on social determinants of health. *BMJ, 341*, c4739. https://doi.org/10.1136/bmj.c4739

Van Den Broucke, S., & Renwart, A. (2014). *La littératie en santé en Belgique: un médiateur des inégalités sociales et des comportements de santé.* Louvain-la-Neuve: Université catholique de Louvain.

Verrept, H. (2012). Notes on the employment of intercultural mediators and interpreters in health care. In D. Ingleby, A. Chiarenza, W. Devillé, & I. Kotsioni (Eds.), *Inequalities in health care for migrants and ethnic minorities* (Vol. 2, pp. 112–127). Antwerpen: Garant.

Whitehead, M., & Dahlgren, G. (2007). *Levelling up (part 1): A discussion paper on concepts and principles for tackling social inequities in health. Studies on social and economic determinants of population health* (Vol. 2). Copenhaguen: WHO Europe.

WHO. (2008). *Health of migrants* (Vol. WHA61.17). Geneva: WHO.

WHO Regional Office for Europe. (2010). *How health systems can address health inequities linked to migration and ethnicity. Briefing policy.* Copenhaguen: WHO Regional Office for Europe.

Chapter 9
Health Policies, Patterns and Barriers to Migrants' Access to Primary Health Care

Sonia Dias, Inês Fronteira, Ana Gama, Andrea Pita Gróz, Deniz Mardin, Jorge Simões, Luis Roxo, and Pedro Pita Barros

9.1 Introduction

As in other countries across the European Union, Portugal has become a destination for an increasing number of migrants from diverse origins in the last decades, which has been a concern for the national agenda (World Health Organization Regional Office for Europe 2014).

Migrants tend to be in relatively good health upon arrival in the host country (Giannoni et al. 2016; Marceca 2017). However, factors such as poor living conditions, socioeconomic disadvantage, undocumented status, and social exclusion have a negative influence on their health over time (Giannoni et al. 2016; Marceca 2017). Being and staying healthy is a fundamental precondition for migrants to work, be productive and contribute to the social and economic development of their communities of origin and destination and is closely linked to integration – illness exacerbates marginalization and marginalization exacerbates illness (Ingleby 2009; International Organization for Migration 2016). Access to good quality health care is an important factor for a good health status and subsequently the social inclusion of migrants (Ingleby 2009).

Developing migrant-friendly policies that address the health dimensions of migration is crucial for the management of health disparities in migrant populations and should address both inequities in the state of health of migrants and in the accessibility and quality of health services available to them (World Health Organization Regional Office for Europe 2010).

S. Dias (✉) · I. Fronteira · A. Gama · A. P. Gróz · J. Simões · L. Roxo · P. P. Barros
Universidade Nova de Lisboa, Lisbon, Portugal
e-mail: smfdias@yahoo.com

D. Mardin
Istanbul University, Istanbul, Turkey

A. Rosano (ed.), *Access to Primary Care and Preventative Health Services of Migrants*, SpringerBriefs in Public Health, https://doi.org/10.1007/978-3-319-73630-3_9

Research has indicated that, even in countries where access to health care is guaranteed, such as Portugal, immigrants do not regularly take advantage of the services available (Almeida et al. 2014; Dias et al. 2011a). A study conducted with 1375 immigrants, in Lisbon, in 2008 concluded that 23% of the participants had never used the National Health Service (NHS) (Dias et al. 2011a). Some of the factors were undocumented status and short length of stay in Portugal. For those who had used the NHS, almost a half sought primary health care (PHC) service in first place, less likely male and undocumented immigrants.

PHC should be a preferential way to access healthcare. PHC offers opportunities for disease prevention and health promotion, and early detection of disease (World Health Organization 2008). In Portugal, PHC has been continuously strengthened with an ongoing reform initiated in 2006 with the purpose of improving the accessibility, proximity, quality and equity of health care, while aiming at satisfying both users and professionals (Ministério da Saúde 2016; World Health Organization 2008).

Portugal faced a financial and economic crisis between 2008 and 2013, with serious social consequences. A number of specific health policy responses to the financial crisis were adopted during this period, namely related to health budget and expenditure cuts, increasing user charges (moderating fees) and changes to health service planning, purchasing and delivery including some measures for PHC (Sakellarides et al. 2014). The context of crisis aggravates economic deprivation and social exclusion, often faced by migrants, placing this population in a situation of greater social vulnerability with impact in access and use of health care services.

Although migrants tend to underuse healthcare services, knowledge about patterns and barriers to access and PHC use is still scarce. In this chapter we explore the existing policies, analyse access and utilization of PHC, describe the main barriers, taking into consideration the PHC reform and the financial crisis.

9.2 Overview of Policies on Access to Health Services and Migration

Over the years, Portugal has been recognized for developing and implementing migrant-friendly policies that promote migrants' access to health services (e.g., endorsement of World Health Assembly resolution WHA61.17 on the health of migrants in May 2008; Table 9.1) (World Health Organization Regional Office for Europe 2014). Portuguese immigration policy is currently guided by Law No. 29/2012 of 9 August 2012, which establishes that immigrants have the same access to the health system as Portuguese citizens (Simões et al. 2017). Foreign citizens are guaranteed the right to be attended in a NHS health centre or hospital, regardless of their nationality, economic means or legal status, once they obtain a health card (or an equivalent document), as defined in the Order no. 25360/2001 of 16 November, issued by the Ministry of Health. In the same Order it is also defined fees exemption

Table 9.1 Timeline overview of the policies on health and migration in Portugal

1976	**Portuguese Constitution** – Recognition of **citizens' right to health care** by "the creation of a universal, free-of-charge **National Health Service**" (NHS)
1989	**Revision of the Portuguese Constitution** "The **National Health Service is universal** and "tendentiously" free of charge, taking into account citizens' social and economic conditions" **Portuguese citizens and legal foreign residents are considered equal** and have similar civil, social and economic rights
1990	**Law no. 48/90 stating the Fundamental Principles of Health** All forms of existing **health care must be made available to everyone** according to needs and irrespective of socio-economic or cultural situation. Health care provided by the NHS includes: health promotion and disease prevention; general and specialized care; nursing care; hospitalization; facultative diagnostic tests; medication and medicinal products; and therapeutic prosthetic devices. Foreign citizens from a third country should have access in reciprocity.
2001	**Order no. 25360/2001** – Specifically concerning **immigrants' access to health services**: Entitlement of foreign citizens to general health care and NHS; Health services cannot refuse treatment based on nationality, lack of economic means, or undocumented status; Full access of undocumented immigrants to NHS after proof of >90 days of residence. Undocumented immigrants are entitled to free care as nationals in situations that jeopardise public health.
2002	Establishment of the High Commissariat for Immigration and Ethnic Minorities, restructured in 2007 into the High Commissariat for Immigration and Intercultural Dialogue (ACIDI, I.P.), presently **High Commission for Migration** (ACM, I.P.).
2004	**Decree-Law no. 67/2004** – National **registry of undocumented children** for their access to health care. **Information Circular no. 65/DSPCS** – Access for **immigrants' children < 16 years to NHS**, independently of legal status.
2006	**Law no. 2/2006, New Nationality Law** – Significant amendments in terms of **acquisition of Portuguese nationality**: Portuguese citizenship accessed by way of nationality of origin or acquisition (adoption or naturalization). Facilitated access to citizenship for immigrants' children born in Portugal.
2007	**Law no. 23/2007, New Immigration Law** – Significant changes in **the conditions for entry, stay and departure** of foreigners into national territory improved considerably the conditions of integration of immigrants into Portuguese society: Any foreign citizen with a valid residence visa for at least 1 year is a legal resident and may apply for a residence permit; Simplified requirements for family reunification; Regime of exception for immigrants showing strong links with Portugal to obtain residence permits; Specific regime for temporary immigration and simplified admission of researchers, academics and highly skilled foreigners; Special regime conceding residence permits to victims of human trafficking and illegal migration. **First Plan for Immigrant Integration (2007–2010)**

(continued)

Table 9.1 (continued)

2009	**Information Circular no. 12/DQS/DMD** – Undocumented immigrants with no document from their parish council certifying that they have been living in Portugal for >90 days are granted access to health care with full payment. Exemptions for specific health situations, children, vaccination, financial needs. Referral to National and/or Local Immigration Support Centres.
2010	**Second Plan for Immigrant Integration (2010–2013)**
2011–2012	**Decree-Laws 113/2011 and 128/2012** – **Fee exemptions** in situations of infectious diseases, pregnancy, children ≤12 years, vaccination, victims of human trafficking, and financial need.
2012	**Law no. 29/2012** – Establishment of the conditions and procedures on the entry, stay, exit and removal of foreign citizens from Portuguese territory, as well as the long-term resident status, with changes to the Law no. 23/2007, namely regarding the Temporary Stay Visa: Validity extended; Increased types of activity included (unpaid professional training, voluntary work or as part of a student exchange programme).
	National Health Plan (2012–2016) – Promotion of **equity and access to health care**, especially among vulnerable groups.
2015	**Strategic Plan for Migration (2015–2020)**

for undocumented migrants in situations that jeopardise public health. In addition, in 2004 it was created a national register of foreign minors who are undocumented and reside in the country, in order to assure their right to health (Decree-Law no. 67/2004).

In 2007, the High Commissariat for Immigration and Intercultural Dialogue (a governmental institution) developed a migrant integration plan that comprised labour and professional training, housing, education and health as areas for action. The main goals were to improve immigrants' knowledge of health care services and promote access to migrant-friendly PHC centres and hospitals. Subsequent plans were developed in 2010 and 2015.

The current National Health Plan also strengthens access of most vulnerable populations to health services, and reinforces PHC services governance and the prioritization of access and quality of PHC.

9.2.1 PHC Reform and Access for Migrants

Under article 64th of the Portuguese Constitution all Portuguese citizens have the right to health, through a NHS tendentiously free at point of delivery, taking into consideration the citizens' economic and social status (Assembleia da República 2005). This means that around 60% of all citizens (including some migrants) pay a small fee (ranging from 4.5 euros for PHC general consultation to 18 euros for general emergency episode) when using NHS services (Simões et al. 2017; The Health Systems and Policy Monitor n.d.). The remaining (chronic patients, children, pregnant women and economic deprived) are exempt from payment (Simões et al. 2017).

Due to the underlying idea of Universal Coverage of the Portuguese NHS, it is considered that migrants, despite their legal status, are entitled to access the NHS. For those who do not hold a residence permit, a document attesting their permanence in Portugal for more than 90 days gives them access to full services of the NHS. Those who are not able to prove residence in Portugal are guaranteed free access in cases of urgent and vital care; communicable diseases (tuberculosis or AIDS, for example); maternal, reproductive and child health care, including family planning, voluntary termination of pregnancy, surveillance of pregnancy, childbirth and childcare, healthcare provided to newborns, and immunization. Irregular migrant children up to 12 years old, foreign citizens in a family reunification situation when someone in the household has proven social security contributions, and patients in a situation of proven economic failure, as well as dependants of their household are also entitled to these services (World Health Organization Regional Office for Europe n.d.).

In Portugal, PHC is the preferred interface between the population and the NHS. In 2006, a PHC reform initiated. Meanwhile, and mainly due to economic crisis, the reform slowed down. This reform aimed at increasing cost-effectiveness of the services while responding to an increasing need for better, more personalized and more responsive healthcare (Simões et al. 2017).

A study conducted in 2016 revealed that 99% of the population is located less than 30 min from a PHC unit (Entidade Reguladora da Saúde 2016) and there is no evidence that this would be different for migrants. Overall, it is considered that the geographical access to PHC of migrants is comparable to that of the general population. However, one can hypothesize that during the financial crisis in Portugal, which had an impact on income and employment, user fees might have had a role in deciding to use services, mainly in non-urgent situations.

Some inequities have been reported in migrants. For instance, higher mortality for all causes, circulatory disease, coronary heart disease, stroke, infectious diseases including AIDS in African migrants when compared to native Portuguese (Harding et al. 2008; Williamson et al. 2009). Also, some differences in sexual and reproductive health have been found in migrants compared to nationals (Campos-Matos et al. 2016).

9.2.2   Access and Use of Health Services

Access and use of health services by migrants in Portugal can be roughly analysed by using data from the National Health Surveys (NHSs) conducted in 2005 (4thNHS) and 2014 (5th NHS). Both included nationals and migrants (defined as born in any country other than Portugal) in a total of 1624 migrants and 33,605 non-migrants, in 2005, and 1331 migrants and 16,871 non-migrants, in 2014. We compared access and use of health services among migrants and non-migrants with ≥15 years of age using data from both surveys (although slight differences exist in some questions of both questionnaires), adjusting for age and sex distribution.

According to data of 2005, migrants were less likely to have a medical appointment in the previous 3 months compared to nationals (aOR = 0.882; IC95 = [0.795;0.979]). No differences were found between migrants and nationals in terms of preventive health behaviours, namely having blood pressure measured (aOR = 0.910; IC95 = [0.717;1.550]) or taking a cholesterol test (aOR = 0.997; IC95 = [0.806; 1.233]) in the last year or having had a mammography in the previous 2 years (aOR = 4.305; IC95 = [0.993;18.652]). However, migrant women between 30 and 60 years were more prone to have pap smear test in the previous 3 years (aOR = 1.950; IC95 = [1.258; 3.024]) compared to national women of the same age group.

In 2014, the chance of having a medical appointment (measured with a specific question about general practice/family medicine consultation in the previous year) was lower among migrants (aOR = 0.911; IC95 = [0.906;0.916]). Migrants were also more likely to not have a health appointment (aOR = 1.360; IC95 = [1.349;1.372]) or buy prescribed medications (OR = 1.074; IC95 = [1.063;1.084]) due to financial problems when compared to nationals (data not available for 2005). Migrants were less likely to have their blood pressure taken (aOR = 0.795; IC95 = [0.791;0.800]), having a cholesterol test (aOR = 0.858; IC95 = [0.853;0.862]) or blood glucose measurement made (aOR = 0.861; IC95 = [0.857;0.866]) when compared to nationals. In 2014, migrant women were less likely to undergo a mammography in the previous 2 years when compared to national women (aOR = 0.500; IC95 = [0.492; 0.508]). Also in 2014, the observed pattern concerning pap smears in 2005 changed and migrant women were less prone to having had a pap smear in the last 3 years (aOR = 0.797; IC95 = [0.789;0.805]). Data from the 5th NHS, in 2014, might corroborate the hypothesis that migrants were probably more affected by financial hardship than nationals, leading to a decrease in their use of preventive and non-urgent medical care, such as mammography or pap smear.

9.2.3 Analysis of Barriers to Access and Use of Health Services

Several studies focus on access and barriers to health services by migrants in Portugal. The majority are qualitative. Barriers depend largely on the type of health services (e.g., preventive medicine) or level of the health system (e.g., PHC). Even among migrants, there are differences depending on gender and source country. However, some of the barriers for migrants are also barriers for nationals (e.g., lack of family doctors, workload of health professionals). We conducted a document analysis to identify some of barriers at organizational, professional and community level, specific to migrants, that impair access to health services in Portugal. An extensive literature review was carried out in PubMed, RCAAP, Google Academics and Scielo for the publications between the years 2000 and 2017. We included in our search peer-reviewed journal articles, thesis and various reports from government and other agencies, all written in Portuguese and English. The legal status of migrants (undocumented or undergoing legalization process) can be an obstacle to access and use of health services in general, and PHC in particular. For instance, difficulties in obtaining a social security number can hamper the access. The social security number is the first information asked by administrative personnel, before contact with health professionals, to register migrants in health services. This number is required by the information system of the health services and without it, migrants cannot be enrolled.

Despite their legal status, migrants should not be excluded from the provision of care, under the Portuguese Law. However, the type of services that they can access to is limited and focused on emergency and urgent situations, sexual and reproductive health and childcare. Migrants mention that many health professionals and administrative personnel are not aware of this, which leads to refusal to deliver healthcare, especially at PHC level. Due to this, migrants tend to access care through emergency departments instead of PHC units. One of the consequences of this pattern is a disruption in continuity of care, which can be particularly relevant in the case of migrants with chronic conditions, women and children.

Another important barrier identified is linked with employment patterns and financial situation. The prevalence of insecure employment (illegal work, lack of contract, agency work) or even unemployment among migrants is high. This places migrants in a very fragile situation in case of illness. Also, the schedules in PHC units are frequently limited to that of "traditional" working hours. For a migrant, attending a medical appointment during work time, even if for pregnancy follow-up or children care, might mean losing a job. This leaves the migrant with either one of two solutions: (1) not attending and thus not accessing appropriate and timely care; or (2) misuse by accessing emergency departments in hospitals (and again failing to have a good follow-up after the illness episode).

Additionally, migrants might not access services because of services fees. Despite most of them being exempt and protected by law, lack of knowledge by migrants might stop them from using services. Also, lack of knowledge by health professionals and administrative personnel might lead them to demand payment when this, in fact, should not be charged.

Still at organizational level, health professionals identify high workload, lack of family doctors, lack of specific training to address migrants' related health and social issues and lack of access to free of charge services as obstacles that migrants have to overcome while accessing health services.

At professional level, one of the barriers is the quality of attendance by health professionals and administrative personnel. Migrants usually feel like second-class citizens, stigmatized and mistreated which leads them only to use health services when absolutely needed, thus impairing preventive medicine, for instance.

Additionally, the inexistence of translators in health services is also a barrier since it impairs an effective communication with consequences in terms of capacity to fully address migrants' health needs and at the same time empowering migrants to effectively manage their health.

On the other hand, insufficient information flows to the migrant community (e.g., on the rights of migrants, available services, social benefits, etc.) are often seen as barriers as they lead to the inability to use effectively the available resources within the health system. Health promotion information is also considered insufficient (and sometimes not culturally appropriate) leaving migrants with less knowledge and capacity to make informed decisions about their health.

At community level, migrants and health professionals point out stigmatisation and non-recognition of the health problem by the community, especially in cases of mental health and HIV infection, as a barrier to access health services. Another aspect pointed out is the frequent lack of information and unawareness of migrants, especially those recently arrived, regarding their health rights and services available. Also, members of the migrants' community mentioned lack of trust in health professionals, fear of being mistreated, fear related to (il)legal status and cost of services as perceived barriers.

9.3   Discussion and Conclusions

In the last decade notorious efforts have been made in Portugal to develop and implement inclusive policies to support immigrants' integration and health promotion. However, empirical evidence shows that many immigrants still tend to underuse the health services, which hinders the provision of timely and adequate health care, especially PHC.

Research conducted so far had shed light on some of the barriers hampering immigrants' access to health services at organizational, professional and community levels. Some of the main barriers in access pointed out by immigrants relate to structural and functioning characteristics of the services (Almeida et al. 2014; Dias et al. 2010). These include cost, strict schedule and highly bureaucratic procedures (Almeida et al. 2014; Dias et al. 2010). Indeed, these constraints have also been documented in previous studies on utilization of healthcare services among Portuguese citizens; however, it tends to disproportionately affect immigrants since often they have less social protection, higher workload and less flexible work schedules (Dias et al. 2008; Fennelly 2004). Even in a context where migrants formally have equal access to healthcare as natives, undocumented immigrants continue to underuse health services, especially for PHC (Dias et al. 2011a; Rodrigues and Schulmann 2014). This is troubling since access to PHC is fundamental in terms of preventive medicine and it is an important health equity indicator.

In times of financial crisis, cost-containment mechanisms, perceived as effective instruments for managing scarce resources, limit the ability of citizens to seek health services, which can result in increased social inequalities (Correia et al. 2017). In the years of the economic crisis, the unmet medical needs increased especially for those unemployed and retired, as well as for those employed citing financial barriers, waiting times, inability to take time off work or family responsibilities as main reasons for not seeking care (Legido-Quigley et al. 2016). Despite scarce research on the effects of financial crisis in immigrants, the described constraints surely also affected this population, that is often socioeconomically more vulnerable. A study on the impact of health system policies resulting from the economic crisis in Portugal showed changes in healthcare seeking behaviour: decrease of 4% in general practitioner appointments, of 28% in PHC urgent attendances and of 9% in hospital emergencies (Sakellarides et al. 2014). PHC visits that did not require a medical consultation increased by 10%, but this increase was only observed for those exempt from user charges (Sakellarides et al. 2014). Nevertheless, more recent data indicate an increase of 0.6% of medical consultations and of 6.9% of nursing consultations at PHC units from 2013 to 2014 (Ministério da Saúde 2015).

With the economic crisis, the increases in unemployment and economic difficulties have rendered many migrants undocumented and created difficulties for proving residency which is connected to difficulties in accessing services (Rodrigues and Schulmann 2014). PHC centres are often wary of granting access to migrants with unclear legal status for fear that they do not pay service fees (Rodrigues and Schulmann 2014). Due to these barriers, migrants often bypass PHC centres, which may indicate that they consequently go directly to hospitals where access is considered to be easier and enforcement of service fees is less stringent (Eurofound 2014). However, when further examinations, treatments or follow-up consultations are required outside the hospital, demanding additional payments, losses of follow-ups and dropouts become common, namely among pregnant women (Rodrigues and Schulmann 2014; Eurofound 2014). Despite the expansion of PHC as recommended in the Memorandum of Understanding agreed upon during the economic crisis, many citizens, especially those from more deprived communities, have experienced barriers accessing PHC, mainly due to increases in co-payments and bureaucratic obstacles (Legido-Quigley et al. 2016). Moreover, cuts in the budget for migrants' health mediators in Portugal, a service specifically designed to improve access by traditionally disadvantaged groups, has contributed to the reduction of the access to care (Eurofound 2014).

In addition to legal and economic constraints in accessing health services, there is still a considerable level of health illiteracy about health rights and access to healthcare among migrants in Portugal. Health professionals are themselves often unaware of migrant rights; this situation has worsened during the period of economic crisis (Almeida et al. 2014; Dias et al. 2010; Eurofound 2014; Rodrigues and Schulmann 2014). A recent study revealed that health professionals and administrative personnel considered to have insufficient knowledge and competencies to deal with culturally diverse immigrant patients, and almost a third was unaware of the legal rights of migrants to access health services (Dias et al. 2011b, 2012).

Presently, the Portuguese economy is showing some signs of improvement. However, it is too soon to know the impact on health. Indeed, many challenges are expected in the coming years and measures are needed to ensure access to care across many population groups including immigrants, in order to mitigate the damage of the recession and the austerity. Although this work focuses on Portugal, considerations can be applied to other similar European countries.

On one hand, further assessment of the impact of the crisis and associated austerity measures on the health of most deprived and vulnerable populations such as immigrants is essential to inform adequate policies and strategies to tackle and minimize negative health effects. Moreover, overcoming the existing barriers in access to health services, especially for PHC, is a crucial step for promoting the health of immigrant populations. In the present financial context, it is fundamental to allocate health resources targeted primarily to those who are most in need. In face of an increasingly diverse population, efforts are needed to continuingly invest in training culturally competent health professionals thus strengthening their capacities to effectively address the health needs of immigrant populations. Another relevant aspect is to improve health literacy among immigrant communities, especially those newly arrived, regarding their health rights, the services available and its functioning characteristics, in order to promote an adequate use of health services, especially for PHC. These recommendations will contribute to promote access to PHC by migrants. Overcoming barriers to and improving quality of health care for migrant populations is key to reduce inequities and consequently to improve health care and obtain health gains for the whole population.

References

Almeida, L. M., Casanova, C., Caldas, J., Ayres-de-Campos, D., & Dias, S. (2014). Migrant women's perceptions of healthcare during pregnancy and early motherhood: Addressing the social determinants of health. *Journal of Immigrant and Minority Health, 16*(4), 719–723. https://doi.org/10.1007/s10903-013-9834-4

Assembleia da República. (2005). Constituição da República Portuguesa – VII Revisão Constitucional (2005). http://www.parlamento.pt/Legislacao/Documents/constpt2005.pdf

Campos-Matos, I., Russo, G., & Perelman, J. (2016). Connecting the dots on health inequalities – a systematic review on the social determinants of health in Portugal. *International Journal for Equity in Health, 15*, 26. https://doi.org/10.1186/s12939-016-0314-z

Correia, T., Carapinheiro, G., Carvalho, H., Silva, J. M., & Vieira, J. (2017). Listening to doctors on patients' use of healthcare during the crisis: Uncovering a different picture and drawing lessons from Portugal. *Journal of Public Health, 39*(2), e56–e62. https://doi.org/10.1093/pubmed/fdw071.

Dias, S., Severo, M., & Barros, H. (2008). Determinants of health care utilization by immigrants in Portugal. *BMC Health Services Research, 8*, 207. https://doi.org/10.1186/1472-6963-8-207

Dias, S., Gama, A., & Rocha, C. (2010). Immigrant women's perceptions and experiences of health care services: Insights from a focus group study. *Journal of Public Health, 18*(5), 489–496. https://doi.org/10.1007/s10389-010-0326-x

Dias, S., Gama, A., Cortes, M., & de Sousa, B. (2011a). Healthcare-seeking patterns among immigrants in Portugal. *Health & Social Care in the Community, 19*(5), 514–521. https://doi.org/10.1111/j.1365-2524.2011.00996.x

Dias, S., Gama, A., Silva, A. C., Cargaleiro, H., & Martins, M. O. (2011b). Barriers in access and utilization of health services among immigrants: The perspective of health professionals. *Acta Médica Portuguesa, 24*(4), 511–516.

Dias, S., Gama, A., Cargaleiro, H., & Martins, M. O. (2012). Health workers' attitudes toward immigrant patients: A cross-sectional survey in primary health care services. *Human Resources for Health, 10*, 14. https://doi.org/10.1186/1478-4491-10-14

Entidade Reguladora da Saúde. (2016). *Estudo sobre as Unidades de Saúde Familiar e as Unidades de Cuidados de Saúde Personalizados* (119 p). Porto: Entidade Reguladora da Saúde. https://www.ers.pt/uploads/writer_file/document/1793/ERS_-_Estudo_USF_e_UCSP_-_final__v.2_.pdf

Eurofound. (2014). *Access to healthcare in times of crisis* (76 p). Luxembourg: Publications Office of the European Union. https://www.eurofound.europa.eu/sites/default/files/ef_publication/field_ef_document/ef1442en.pdf

Fennelly, K. (2004). *Listening to the experts: Provider recommendations on the health needs of immigrants and refugees*. Malmo: Malmo University.

Giannoni, M., Franzini, L., & Masiero, G. (2016). Migrant integration policies and health inequalities in Europe. *BMC Public Health, 16*, 463. https://doi.org/10.1186/s12889-016-3095-9

Harding, S., Teyhan, A., Rosato, M., & Santana, P. (2008). All cause and cardiovascular mortality in African migrants living in Portugal: Evidence of large social inequalities. *European Journal of Cardiovascular Prevention and Rehabilitation, 15*(6), 670–676. https://doi.org/10.1097/HJR.0b013e32830fe6ce

Ingleby, D. (2009). *European research on migration and health. Background paper* (18 p). Geneva: International Organization for Migration. http://www.migrant-health-europe.org/files/UUIngleby%20&%20IOM%20Peiro_Day%201_Session%202_24_09.pdf

International Organization for Migration. (2016). *Migration health – annual review 2015* (112 p). Geneva: International Organization for Migration. https://publications.iom.int/system/files/mhd_ar_2015.pdf

Legido-Quigley, H., Karanikolos, M., Hernandez-Plaza, S., de Freitas, C., Bernardo, L., Padilla, B., et al. (2016). Effects of the financial crisis and Troika austerity measures on health and health care access in Portugal. *Health Policy, 120*(7), 833–839. https://doi.org/10.1016/j.healthpol.2016.04.009

Marceca, M. (2017). Migration and health from a public health perspective. In I. Muenstermann (Ed.), *People's movements in the 21st century – risks, challenges and benefits* (pp. 103–127). Rijeka: InTech.

Ministério da Saúde. (2015). *Relatório anual sobre o acesso a cuidados de saúde nos estabelecimentos do SNS e entidades convencionadas (2014)* (114 p). Ministério da Saúde: Lisboa. https://www.sns.gov.pt/wp-content/uploads/2016/07/2015-07-20-RA_Acesso_2014-VFinal.pdf

Ministério da Saúde. (2016). *Reforma do Serviço Nacional de Saúde – Coordenação nacional para os Cuidados de Saúde Primários. Plano Estratégico e Operacional* (6 p). Ministério da Saúde: Lisboa. https://www.sns.gov.pt/wp-content/uploads/2016/02/Plano_Estrategico_e_Operacional.pdf

Rodrigues, R., & Schulmann, K. (2014). *Impacts of the crisis on access to healthcare services: Country report on Portugal* (51 p). European Centre for Social Welfare Policy and Research: Wien. http://www.euro.centre.org/data/1402559638_38546.pdf

Sakellarides, C., Castelo-Branco, L., Barbosa, P., & Azevedo, H. (2014). *The impact of the financial crisis on the health system and health in Portugal* (44 p). Copenhagen: World Health Organization. http://www.euro.who.int/__data/assets/pdf_file/0006/266388/The-impact-of-the-financial-crisis-on-the-health-system-and-health-in-Portugal.pdf?ua=1

Simões, J. A., Augusto, G. F., Fronteira, I., & Hernández-Quevedo, C. (2017). Portugal: Health system review. *Health Systems in Transition, 19*(2), 1–184.

The Health Systems and Policy Monitor. (n.d.). *Country page for Portugal*. http://www.hspm.org/countries/portugal25062012/countrypage.aspx. Accessed 20 June 2017.

Williamson, L. M., Rosato, M., Teyhan, A., Santana, P., & Harding, S. (2009). AIDS mortality in African migrants living in Portugal: Evidence of large social inequalities. *Sexually Transmitted Infections, 85*(6), 427–431. https://doi.org/10.1136/sti.2008.034066

World Health Organization. (2008). *The world health report. Primary health care – now more than ever* (119 p). Geneva: World Health Organization. http://www.who.int/whr/2008/whr08_en.pdf

World Health Organization Regional Office for Europe. (2010). *How health systems can address health inequities linked to migration and ethnicity* (35 p). Copenhagen: WHO Regional Office for Europe. http://www.euro.who.int/__data/assets/pdf_file/0005/127526/e94497.pdf

World Health Organization Regional Office for Europe. (2014). *Portugal: Assessing health-system capacity to manage sudden large influxes of migrants* (10 p). Copenhagen: WHO Regional Office for Europe. http://www.euro.who.int/__data/assets/pdf_file/0016/265012/Portugal-assessing-health-system-capacity-to-manage-sudden-large-influxes-of-migrants.pdf

World Health Organization Regional Office for Europe. (n.d.). *Migration and health: key issues*. http://www.euro.who.int/en/health-topics/health-determinants/migration-and-health/migrant-health-in-the-european-region/migration-and-health-key-issues#292117. Accessed 26 Nov 2016.

Concluding Remarks

Over these last decades, there is an increasing interest on migrant health, especially regarding how migrant health issues affect the individuals and the populations but also the overall society, from local level to global level, including health policies, health care costs and efficient use of resources. In that sense, prevention has a key role to ensure the sustainability and the efficiency of the health care system. This book provides an accurate and up-to-date information on the access to preventive health services of migrants in the European region. This description is completed with the most recent evidences from all around the world such as the USA, Australia and European countries with a long or recent history of taking care of migrants.

Access to PHS for migrants' access is affected differently at different levels of the health system: migrants have often a lower access to PHS when compared to nationals. Several issues are concerned with equity in health care access, such as entitlement, health policies, structure and organization of services, and the attitude of health professionals towards migrants. A major finding of this book is that, even in countries with a favourable legal framework of entitlement, migrants encounter difficulties in accessing PHS, supporting the need for more actions to help them to gain access to quality PHS. Lack of targeted policies may partly explain the large gap between nationals and migrants in accessing PHS, as well as the lack of training of health care professionals. Moreover, among the multitude of factors affecting access to PHS, migrants encounter peculiar hurdles such as linguistic and cultural problems and lack of access to information, affecting the poorly educated and those with a poor health literacy. Differences in cultural beliefs and languages make it even more difficult for service providers to meet the needs of migrants. Attributes other than migration status, such as sexual orientation or gender identity further complicate access to health care, specifically when diversity management is not part of the health policy agenda. This may lead to poor perceptions and attitudes of individual health care professionals providing services for migrants. Improving access will thus require a whole-health-system approach, from the patients to the political level.

© The Author(s), under exclusive licence to Springer International Publishing AG, part of Springer Nature 2018
A. Rosano (ed.), *Access to Primary Care and Preventative Health Services of Migrants*, SpringerBriefs in Public Health, https://doi.org/10.1007/978-3-319-73630-3

Health policies may facilitate the access of migrants to health services by defining entitlements by law, publicizing them to migrants and health care providers and ensuring appropriate implementation measures but need to be sustainable, implemented and provided with adequate human and material resources.

Index

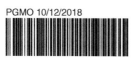